1994 Edition

Managed Care Desk Reference

The Complete Guide to Terminology and Resources

A convenient desktop resource containing a comprehensive glossary and up-to-date information sources covering the entire managed care industry

Marianne F. Fazen, Ph.D.

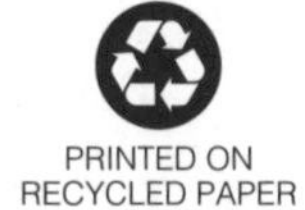

Managed Care Desk Reference, 1994 Edition
by Marianne F. Fazen, Ph.D.

97 96 95 94 4 3 2 1

Publisher:	HCS Publications
Composition Consultant:	Russ Mauch Innovative Resource Systems Co.
Book Design:	Gordon Cathey Cathey Associates, Inc.
Production:	The Graphics Group
Production Manager:	Joyce Day

ISBN: 0-9639835-0-4

To my children,
Stephen and his wife, Lynn,
and Michael

About the Author

Marianne F. Fazen, Ph.D. is president of HealthCare Strategies, a strategic management firm which she founded in 1990. Dr. Fazen also is an adjunct professor at the University of Dallas, teaching strategic health care marketing to graduate students, and a frequent speaker and contributor to professional publications.

Prior to starting her consulting business, Dr. Fazen worked for Voluntary Hospitals of America, Inc., initially as manager of market research and later, as manager of managed care research and information. She is active in several professional associations, including the Society for Healthcare Planning and Marketing, the Dallas/Fort Worth Managed Care Forum, and the American Marketing Association. She has been a member of the Board of Directors of the local American Marketing Association Chapter for six years and is a co-founder of the Chapter's Health Care Section.

Dr. Fazen received her undergraduate degree in Medical Technology from the University of Wisconsin and her doctorate in Communications Science and Human Development from University of Texas at Dallas.

Acknowledgments

A project like this is never the work of only the author. If it were not for the assistance, support and encouragement of many people, this book would not have been written.

I am deeply indebted to Dr. Lynn Eckhert, professor and chairman of the Department of Family and Community Medicine at the University of Massachusetts, and to Bill Lewis, medical economics analyst for Kaiser Permanente, for meticulously reviewing the definitions and offering countless points of advice on improving the presentation of the material. The physician's perspective provided by Dr. Eckhert and Mr. Lewis' knowledge of the managed care business ensured the accuracy of this work.

Dr. Kathleen Griffin, founding chairman of the board of the International Subacute Healthcare Association, deserves credit for sparking the idea for this undertaking nearly a year ago when she asked me to prepare a brief glossary of managed care terms for the American Speech-Language and Hearing Association (ASHA). The brief version for ASHA became the springboard for the broad-based, comprehensive collection of terms contained in the ***Managed Care Desk Reference.***

I am also grateful to Pat Crosetti, vice president of VHA Mid-America, and Kendra Fuller, director of sales for Anthem Health Systems, Inc., whose experience with hospitals, integrated health care systems, and managed care organizations ensured that the terms used by these key stakeholder groups were accurately defined and clearly presented.

The technical advice generously provided by Susan Alt, president of The Business Word, Inc., regarding the publishing business helped me avoid mistakes and saved me many times over from reinventing the wheel.

Finally, the person deserving my deepest appreciation and gratitude is my husband, Robert, whose unfaltering support, patience, and understanding gave me the determination and persistence to see this project through to completion and make this book a reality.

"The finest words in the world are only vain sounds, if you cannot comprehend them."

Anatole France (1844 - 1924)

Preface

Communication is either a bridge or a barrier. As a bridge, it is built with commonly-understood words that create insight, awareness, and consensus. As a barrier, it is erected with arcane, vague, or uniquely-defined terminology that creates misunderstanding, distrust and separation. This duality of communication is particularly troublesome in the evolving field of managed health care.

As it has spread throughout the United States, managed care has been embraced by an expanding array of groups. Each group—employers, employees, insurance companies, health care providers, government agencies, labor unions, etc.—understandably has its own concerns and perceptions. But each group also has its own terminology for expressing these concerns and perceptions. When this terminology is not shared—or worse, not understood!—by the other groups with a stake in managed care, potential communication bridges quickly become communication barriers.

The ***Managed Care Desk Reference*** resolves this problem by providing a common reference point for managed care terminology. Past and current terms are defined using context-based definitions. This type of definition not only identifies what a term means, but demonstrates how it is used in a managed care context. Acronyms are also presented and defined so that mysterious phrases, like "the ADL exceeds the MAP specified in the COC," can be accurately interpreted and understood. A comprehensive glossary eliminates time-wasting searches, and extensive cross-referencing places collateral information at the user's fingertips.

The ***Managed Care Desk Reference*** is really two resources in one. In addition to the comprehensive glossary of terms, it includes a list of organizations, agencies and associations in the forefront of managed care development, delivery, management, accreditation, review, policy formulation, and research. Complete contact information is provided in convenient, tabbed sections.

Every aspect of the ***Managed Care Desk Reference*** has been designed with practicality and user convenience in mind. From its no-nonsense definitions and easy-to-read print, to its fully indexed layout and convenient size, the ***Managed Care Desk Reference*** offers quick and easy access to current managed care terminology and usage. Annual revisions will ensure that the information in the ***Managed Care Desk Reference*** remains current.

Although the objective of managed care is straightforward, that is, to provide high quality, patient-centered health care that is both accessible and cost-effective, the terminology to achieve this objective has not been. With the ***Managed Care Desk Reference,*** providers, purchasers, payors and patients will at last have the resource they need to speak the same language. As a result, health care stakeholders can focus their attention on issues rather than on semantics, and ensure that the objective of managed care is fully realized.

M.Fazen
1/3/94

Explanatory Notes

Terms in this book have been selected from numerous sources, including textbooks, trade publications, professional journals and government publications. The aim was to bring together in a single desktop resource the wide variety of specialized terminology and jargon used by managed care stakeholders from many different industries and the key organizations involved in various aspects of managed health care financing, delivery and management.

Alphabetization
Terms are listed alphabetically and printed in boldface type. If a term is commonly known by its abbreviation or acronym, the abbreviation or acronym is shown in parentheses immediately following the term. Abbreviations and acronyms are also separately listed alphabetically in their own section (**Part I, Section 2**).

Many terms in this book have more than one meaning. In most cases, only the meaning relating to managed care is provided. For example, the term a*ppeal* may mean "to take a case to a higher court," or "to plead for help," or "to arouse a sympathetic response." In the language of managed care, *appeal* means "to request a claims processor to reconsider a determination not to certify an admission, extension of stay, or other health care service." This is the definition given in this book.

Part I—Managed Care Terminology

Related Terms
Many of the entries in **Part I** include one or more related terms which the user may want to review to obtain a broader understanding of the topics. For easy cross-referencing, related terms appear directly below the main entry, following the directive, "*See also.*"

Often, the related term may be used in the definition. Occasionally, however, when a term isa closely related concept or provides contrast, it is cross-referenced, even though it is not used in the definition. When a related term is used in the definition, it is printed in italics only the first time it appears in the definition.

Cross References
When an entry is merely another expression for a term defined elsewhere in the book, a cross-reference rather than a definition is provided. In the example, "**Factored Rating**—See: **Adjusted Community Rating**," the reader is directed to another expression of the same concept where the definition may be found.

Part II—Information Resources

Generally, information about the organizations listed in the **Information Resources** sections of **Part II** was provided by the organizations themselves. In some cases, information was obtained from other published sources. In all cases, contact information was verified with the respective organizations to ensure that what appears in this reference guide is current and accurate.

An attempt was made by the author to include organizations that are at the forefront of managed health care financing, delivery, management, accreditation, policy formulation, and research. The reader is urged to bring to the author's attention any organizations which the reader believes should be included. Consideration will be given to readers' suggestions for the next edition of the ***Managed Care Desk Reference.***

A Note Regarding Comprehensiveness

One of the main objectives in preparing the ***Managed Care Desk Reference*** was to make this book as comprehensive as possible, given that the number of terms used in managed care is very large, and constantly growing. The author has attempted thoroughness in determining which terms belong in this book, but is aware that not all terms have been included. The reader is asked to regard any exclusions as either editorial decisions or oversights by the author.

Readers are encouraged to bring to the author's attention any terms or names of organizations that the reader thinks should be included. Also, the author welcomes any comments regarding the definitions, which the reader believes will improve the ***Managed Care Desk Reference.***

1994 Edition

Managed Care Desk Reference

The Complete Guide to Terminology and Resources

Book Sections

Section 1
Terms

All terms in the following section are listed alphabetically. In cases where a term is also known by its acronym or abbreviation, the acronym or abbreviation appears in parentheses after the term. Related and collateral terms that provide additional information or contrast are listed as *"see also"* terms.

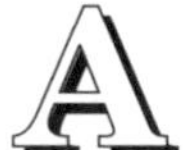

Academy of Managed Care Pharmacy (AMCP)

A national professional society of pharmacists, organized for the purpose of promoting the development and advancement of pharmaceutical care in managed health care environments. The AMCP had 1700 members in 1993, representing approximately 200 managed care organizations. AMCP provides educational programs, including two annual national conferences and several regional conferences, bimonthly newsletters, and other resources useful to members. AMCP also monitors legislative issues that impact managed care pharmacy and is proactive in the development of position statements and related resource materials.
Address: AMCP, 1321 Duke Street, Suite 305, Alexandria, VA 22314
Phone: (703) 683-8416 or (800) TAP-AMCP
Fax: (703) 683-8417

Access

See also:
Universal Access

Refers to the patient's ability to obtain medical care. Ease of access is determined by a number of factors, such as availability of medical services and their acceptability to the patient, location of health care facilities, transportation, hours of operation, cost of care, languages spoken by both patients and providers, and socio-cultural beliefs and attitudes.

Accountable Health Partnership (AHP)

See also:
Standard Benefits Package;
Jackson Hole Group (JHG);
Managed Competition

Under the proposed *managed competition* model for health care reform developed by the *Jackson Hole Group,* an "accountable health partnership" (AHP) would consist of an insurer and health care provider working separately or collaboratively to provide health care benefits and services within a geographical area. "Qualified AHPs" would be certified that they meet underwriting standards and can deliver a *standard benefits package* in accordance with generally accepted health care accounting practices. Tax-advantaged premiums for employers and individuals would be available only through qualified AHPs.

Accreditation

See also:
American Accreditation Program, Inc. (AAPI);
National Committee for Quality Assurance (NCQA);
Utilization Review Accreditation Commission (URAC)

A standardized program for evaluating a health care organization to ensure a specified level of quality, as defined by a set of industry standards. Organizations that meet accreditation criteria receive an official authorization of approval of their products and services. The accreditation process is designed to be non-confrontational and educational. It provides the organization an opportunity to evaluate its operations and systems, and compare its products and services to state-of-the-art products and services. Increasingly, accreditation of managed care organizations is becoming a requirement by purchasers and payors for participation in managed care plans.

Accrete

See also:
Accrual;
Delete

A term used by Medicare to describe the process of adding new enrollees to a health plan. In non-health care industries, the term *accrete* may be used synonymously with *accrue* in accounting practice. In managed care, however, *accrete* is an enrollment term and *accrue* is a financial term. The antonym for acrete is *delete*.

Accrual

See also:
Claims Reserve

An accounting method used by managed care plans in which medical expenses of enrollees are estimated for a given period, usually ending at the financial month closing. The accrual method uses a combination of data from various information sources, such as authorization data, claims history, lag studies, etc. Funds are then set aside in a *claims reserve* to be used for medical expenses as incurred during that period.

Activities of Daily Living (ADL)

See also:
Health Status

The normal activities performed as a part of a person's daily routine of self-care. Examples of ADL include: bathing, dressing, eating, continence, etc. ADLs are often used as indicators of a patient's *health status* following medical treatment or hospitalization.

Actuarial Assumptions

See also:
Actuary

The assumptions that an *actuary* uses in calculating the expected costs and revenues of a managed care plan. Utilization rates, age and sex, enrollee mix, cost for medical services, etc. are examples of actuarial assumptions.

Actuary

See also:
Actuarial Assumptions

An insurance professional who has been trained to apply probability and statistics to determine policy premiums, calculate reserves and dividends, perform financial forecasts and other statistical studies. Actuaries often advise in situations involving questions of probability.

Acute Care

See also:
Chronic Care;
Long-Term Care

Treatment for a short-term or episodic illness or health problem (as opposed to a *chronic* or long-term illness).

Adjudication

See also:
Formal Grievance Procedure

The formal process of making a decision on a claim or resolving a disputed claim in claims administration. The number of adjudicators on a claims administration team usually depends on the volume and type of claims received. For example, an HMO might hire one adjudicator for every 8,000 to 10,000 members.

Adjusted Average Per Capital Cost (AAPCC)

See also:
Average Payment Rate (APR)

The estimated average cost of providing health care services to Medicare beneficiaries in a specified geographical area. The AAPCC is based on the following factors: age, sex, institutional status, Medicaid, disability and end stage renal disease status. HCFA uses AAPCCs to calculate monthly Medicare payments both to Medicare Risk and cost-based providers under contract.

Adjusted Community Rating (ACR)

See also:
Community Rating; Experience Rating

A rate-setting methodology used by many managed care plans for prospectively determining group rates for each group's expected use of health care services during an upcoming contract period (usually one year). The ACR is based on a group's prior use of health care services. In other words, past trends are used to determine the group's future use of services relative to the average use for all members. This is the "adjustment factor" which is then applied (i.e., multiplied) to the basic community rates, yielding "adjusted community rates." The adjusted community rates then represent the expected revenue required to provide services to group members during the contract period. The group's rate is fixed for that period and is not subject to retroactive adjustment to reflect the group's actual use of health services. Sometimes called *factored rating*.

Administrative Costs

See also:
National Health Expenditures (NHE); Retention

Refers to costs associated with various administrative functions of providers and payors, including transaction-related costs, benefit management costs, insurance marketing and selling costs, taxes, and costs associated with compliance with government regulations. In government estimates of *national health expenditures (NHE),* administrative costs are defined as the costs of administering government health benefits programs (Medicare, Medicaid) plus the net cost of private insurance. Administrative costs associated with health care are difficult to define and accurately measure because these costs are fluid, shifting from one sector (insurers, hospitals, physicians, employers, consumers, etc.) to another depending on the benefit design, insurance system, or method of claims processing. Also called *retention.*

Administrative Services Only Contract (ASO)

See also:
Self-Funded Plan; Third Party Administrator (TPA)

A contract between an independent agent, such as an insurance company or *third party administrator (TPA),* and a *self-funded plan* whereby the agent performs administrative services only and does not assume any potential financial liability (i.e., "risk"). ASO services typically include claims processing and other administrative functions. Other services, such as actuarial analysis and utilization review, may also be included.

Admissions (Admits)

See also:
Admissions/1000; Discharges

The number of patients placed (i.e., "admitted") in a hospital or inpatient facility for an overnight stay per given time period. The term usually refers to hospitalizations, but may also refer to inpatients in an extended care facility. The antonym is *discharges.*

Admissions/1000

See also:
Admissions (Admits); Member Months

An inpatient volume measure indicating the number of hospital *admissions* per 1,000 members of a defined population. Health plans use this measure to indicate and/or estimate use rates for various inpatient services. The formula used by health plans for calculating admissions/1000 is: number of admissions per *member months* times 1000 members times the number of months.

Adult Day Care

See also:
Activities of Daily Living (ADL)

A range of services, such as health, medical, psychological, social, nutritional and educational services, provided during the day on a regular basis, allowing an adult to live at home rather than in an institution. Adult day care centers are usually targeted toward seniors who do not need around-the-clock nursing care, but require assistance performing the basic *activities of daily living (ADL)*. These centers offer a lower cost alternative to families other than nursing homes and often provide a family member with a necessary transitional stage prior to entry into a nursing home. Adult day care is usually not covered by health insurance policies or managed care plans.

Advance Practice Nurse (APN)

See: **Nurse Practitioner (NP)**

Adverse Selection

See also:
Community Rating

A situation which occurs when a managed care plan attracts members who are sicker or more likely to use more and costlier services than the general population. Adverse selection tends to be a problem for managed care plans, particularly HMOs, that use *community rating* for setting rates. It becomes an expensive problem for managed care plans if some members are sicker or have a potential for higher health care utilization (i.e., "high risk") than was anticipated when the budget for medical costs was being determined. Adverse selection can also be a problem when a plan does not screen for pre-existing conditions.

After-Hours Care

See also:
Call Schedule;
Out-of-Network Services (OON)

Medical services requested or required when an outpatient facility, such as an HMO clinic, is not open. After-hours care may consist of a telephone referral to a managed care plan's own emergency unit or to another facility outside of its network (*out-of-network services*).

Aftercare

See also:
Discharge Planning

Individualized medical services provided to patients following hospitalization or rehabilitation according to arrangements made through the *discharge planning* program. The objective of aftercare is to gradually phase the patient out of treatment while providing follow-up attention to prevent relapse.

Against Medical Advice

See also:
Discharge Status

A *discharge status* assigned to a patient who leaves the hospital against the advice of his/her physician or the medical staff. Normally in such a case, the patient is asked to sign a release of the hospital and attending physician from responsibility. Occasionally, a patient leaves the hospital without the knowledge of hospital personnel and also is classified as discharged "against medical advice."

Age/Sex Rates (ASR)

See also:
Table Rates

A table of rates used for setting rates for a group health plan in which separate rates are listed for each grouping of age and sex categories. ASRs are used to calculate premiums for group billing purposes. For small groups, this type of premium structure is usually preferred over single and family ratings because it automatically adjusts to demographic changes in the group. Also called *table rates*.

Agency for Health Care Policy and Research (AHCPR)

An agency of the U. S. Public Health Service within the Department of Health & Human Services (HHS), which funds and conducts health services research and assessments of health care technologies. ACHPR programs focus on: 1) development, publication, and dissemination of clinical practice guidelines and information for patients (in English and Spanish); 2) medical treatment effectiveness studies, including 14 Patient Outcomes Research Teams (PORTs), which assess alternative methods for diagnosing, treating, managing, or preventing a particular condition; 3) evaluation of risks, benefits, and effectiveness of new or unestablished medical devices, procedures, and other health care technologies; 4) programs that address access to health services, cost, financing, and quality of care. The agency offers numerous publications through its AHCPR Publications Clearinghouse that describe its programs and present research findings and technology assessments.
Address: AHCPR, 2101 E. Jefferson St., Suite 501, Rockville, MD 20852
Phone: (800) 358-9295; Fax: (301) 594-2283

Alcoholism Program

See also:
Detoxification;
Substance Abuse

Activities, services and functions (including alcohol abuse education) connected with the planning, direction, or coordination of treatment and rehabilitation of the alcoholic or the prevention of alcoholism. Alcoholism programs may be inpatient or outpatient.

All Clause Deductible

See also:
Deductible

A *deductible* applied to all covered expenses incurred by a plan member as a result of the same or related causes within a given time period, called the "accumulation time."

All Payers System

See also:
Third Party Payor

A rate-setting program used by some providers that subjects all *third party payors*, including both public and private payers, to the same rules of reimbursement as a condition of contracting with the payers.

Allied Health Professional

See also:
Certified Nurse Midwife (CNM);
Nurse Practitioner (NP);
Physician's Assistant (PA)

A specially trained and licensed (when necessary) health care worker other than a physician, dentist, optometrist, podiatrist, or chiropractor. Allied health professionals include: paramedics, *physician's assistants (PA), certified nurse midwives (CNM), nurse practitioners (NP),* and other caregivers who perform tasks that otherwise would be performed by a physician. Allied health professionals usually work under the supervision of a physician and provide care at a lower cost. Also called *medical assistant (MA).*

Allocated Benefits

See also:
Maximum Allowable Payment (MAP);
Unallocated Benefits

Benefits for which the *maximum allowable payment (MAP)* under a health plan for specific services is itemized in the insurance or managed care contract. (Contrast with *unallocated benefits.*)

Allopathic

See also:
Homeopathic;
Osteopathic

A system of therapy in which diseases are treated by producing a condition in the patient that is incompatible with or antagonistic to the condition to be cured. Allopathic physicians, which comprise most of the physicians in the United States, as distinguished from *osteopathic* and *homeopathic* physicians, view the role of the physician as an active interventionist who attempts to counteract the effects of disease by using surgical or medical treatments that produce effects opposite to those of the disease. Allopathic medicine also incorporates a preventive approach to health care.

Allowable Costs

See also:
Certificate of Coverage (COC);
Covered Expenses

Charges for medical services or supplies provided by a hospital or physician which qualify as *covered expenses* as stated in the health plan's *certificate of coverage (COC).*

Alpha Center

See also:
Robert Wood Johnson Foundation (RWJF)

A private, non-profit health policy organization, which sponsors demonstration and research programs, facilitates changes in health care financing and organization, provides technical assistance and guidance on health policy issues, and disseminates policy and research results through briefings and publications targeted to national audiences. Alpha Center directs the "Health Care for the Uninsured Program" and the "Changes in Health Care Financing and Organization" initiatives for the *Robert Wood Johnson Foundation (RWJF)*. The organization also conducts educational conferences and workshops on health policy and planning topics, provides a resource center and library for information on a wide variety of health-related topics, and distributes a newsletter, Health Care for the Uninsured Program Update.
Address: Alpha Center, 1350 Connecticut Ave., NW, Suite 1100, Washington, DC 20036
Phone: (202) 296-1818; Fax: (202) 296-1825

Alternative Delivery Systems (ADS)

See also:
Coordinated Care; Managed Care

A term used during the 1980s and before to describe non-traditional methods of providing health benefits. Usually that meant non-indemnity insurance-based methods. ADS has been replaced by the term *managed care* to describe health care delivery and financing systems that limit provider selection and incorporate utilization management and cost control techniques. The term *coordinated care* emerged in the health care lexicon during the Bush Administration to describe alternative delivery systems, or managed care. Regardless of the popularity of one term over another, they all refer to health care financing and delivery systems and processes for providing medically necessary services in a more cost-effective manner than traditional indemnity insurance-based methods.

Alternative Therapies

See also:
Alternative Treatment Benefit Provision

Unconventional or non-standard treatments for illnesses or health conditions that are considered to be outside mainstream medicine. Examples of alternative therapies include: relaxation techniques, massage, biofeedback, yoga, hypnosis, imagery, homeopathy, naturopathy, chiropractic, acupuncture, spiritual healing, weight-loss programs, macrobiotics and other lifestyle diets, herbal medicine, megavitamins, self-help groups, energy healing, and folk remedies. It is estimated that one-third of Americans seek relief through alternative therapies and spend nearly $14 billion a year on such treatments. Some managed care plans have an *alternative treatment benefit provision,* which allows consideration of alternative therapies if deemed appropriate for the patient's presenting condition. Several alternative therapies, such as massage therapy, yoga, and acupuncture and music therapy, are now receiving federal funds from the National Institutes of Health's newly established (in January, 1993) Office of Alternative Medicine for study by conventional scientific methods.

Alternative Treatment Benefit Provision

See also:
Alternative Therapies

A benefit available in some health plans that gives consideration to professionally accepted *alternative therapies*, procedures, services, or courses of treatment that might be performed (often at a lower cost) to accomplish the desired outcome.

Ambulatory Care

See also:
Free-Standing Outpatient Surgery Center;
Outpatient Care;
Primary Care Physician / Practitioner (PCP)

Health care services provided to patients who are able to return home without an overnight stay in a medical facility. Typically, ambulatory care includes preventive, diagnostic, and treatment services provided on an outpatient basis, for example, at medical offices, *free-standing outpatient surgery centers,* or other types of outpatient clinics by either physicians, surgeons, or non-physician *primary care practitioners* (e.g., nurse practitioners, physician's assistants). Ambulatory care services tend to be less costly than inpatient hospital care and are usually favored by managed care plans. Also known as *outpatient care.*

Ambulatory Patient Group (APG)

See also:
Ambulatory Care;
Ancillary Services;
Diagnosis-Related Group (DRG);
Outpatient

An outpatient case-mix reimbursement methodology which groups patients according to clinical characteristics, resource use, and costs. Procedures provided in the hospital outpatient setting are classified by APGs in a way similar to the DRG classification system for hospital inpatient procedures. Objectives of the APG system are to establish a fixed reimbursement system for outpatient procedures and visits, incorporate patient data and information regarding the reason for the *outpatient* visit, and prevent unbundling of *ancillary services*. The APG classification system was developed for HCFA by 3M Health Information Systems, an independent MIS vendor.

American Academy of Family Physicians (AAFP)

See also:
Family Practice (FP)

A professional society for physicians in *family practice (FP),* of which 65% provide care to patients enrolled in a managed care plan, according to a 1991 member survey. AAFP helps FP physicians interact effectively with managed care organizations and succeed in this important and growing segment of their practices. The organization monitors managed care trends, develops policy and programming in this regard, and holds an annual managed care-focused conference.
Address: AAFP, 8880 Ward Parkway,
Kansas City, MO 64114
Phone: (816) 333-9700; Fax: (816) 822-0580

American Accreditation Program, Inc. (AAPI)

See also:
Accreditation;
American Association of Preferred Provider Organizations (AAPPO)

A corporation which offers an *accreditation* program for PPOs seeking an endorsement of their products in the marketplace. The AAPI was created by the *American Association of Preferred Provider Organizations (AAPPO)* in 1989 in response to criticism of PPOs by health care purchasers and industry competitors. Unlike HMOs, PPOs are not federally regulated, and state-level regulation varies considerably. AAPI has developed a set of eight criteria, or *standards*, that define a managed care PPO: 1) network; 2) legal structure; 3) provider selection; 4) utilization management; 5) administration capabilities; 6) financial solvency; 7) quality assessment; and 8) payment methodologies. Medicare and some large employers both have used AAPI's protocols as a basis for selecting and contracting with PPOs. "Pure discount" PPO networks are not considered "managed care" by the AAPI, and therefore, are not eligible for its accreditation program.
Address: AAPI, 2270 Cedar Cove Court,
Reston, VA 22091
Phone: (703) 860-5900; Fax: (703) 860-5901

A

American Association of Physician-Hospital Organizations (AAPHO)

See also:
Physician-Hospital Organization (PHO)

A recently established (in 1993) national organization which serves as a resource for networking, education and advocacy for physicians, hospitals, and *Physician-Hospital Organizations (PHO)* interested in furthering the development of PHOs. Creation of the AAPHO was spearheaded by executives at the Piedmont Healthcare Organization, a PHO affiliated with Piedmont Hospital in Atlanta, GA. Its first symposium has been scheduled for February 10-11, 1994, in Atlanta, GA. Additional educational conferences are planned throughout the year. AAPHO publications include a quarterly newsletter (AAPHO Insights), a membership directory, and a consultants directory. The AAPHO also offers members preferred rates for consultants.
Address: AAPHO, P. O. Box 4913, Glen Allen, VA 23058-4913
Phone: (800) 722-0376; Fax: (804) 747-5316

American Association of Preferred Provider Organizations (AAPPO)

See also:
Preferred Provider Organization (PPO)

A national trade organization representing *preferred provider organizations (PPO)* and their partners in managed care. Members include PPOs, insurance companies, physicians, hospitals, consultants, TPAs, and pharmaceutical companies. The AAPPO's mission is to provide direction and assistance to and for the managed healthcare industry through education, information, research, and advocacy. Membership benefits include: national conferences, regional seminars, publications (e.g., Directory of Operational PPOs), research activities, and networking opportunities. The AAPPO represents its members' views to the trade and media, monitors the legislative and regulatory environment, and advocates PPOs and related issues at national, state, and local levels.
Address: AAPPO, 1101 Connecticut Ave., Suite 700, Washington, DC 20036
Phone: (202) 429-5133; Fax: (202) 429-5108

American Federation of Home Health Agencies (AFHHA)

See also:
Home Healthcare Agency (HHA);
Visiting Nurse Association of America (VNAA)

A national trade organization representing the interests of Medicare-certified *home healthcare agencies (HHA)* in legislative and regulatory processes. Membership includes a variety of home health providers, including free-standing, hospital-based, and chain HHAs, *visiting nurse association (VNA)* agencies, and county agencies. Membership also is open to state home health associations, vendors, consultants, and individuals. Its primary objective is to influence public policy processes. AFHHA monitors national legislative developments, provides technical advice and support, educational seminars, and networking opportunities to members. Publications include the Insider newsletter, and legislative and regulatory "alerts."
Address: AFHHA, 1320 Fenwick Lane, Suite 100, Silver Spring, MD 20910
Phone: (301) 588-1454; Fax: (301) 588-4732

A

American Health Care Association (AHCA)

See also:
Long-Term Care (LTC)

A national federation of 51 associations (in 1993) representing 11,000 non-profit and for-profit *long- term care (LTC)* providers. AHCA promotes standards for LTC professionals and quality care for LTC residents. AHCA provides members information on legislative and regulatory policy and initiatives, health care management, facility administration, and pertinent products and services through its monthly publication, Provider, and biweekly newsletter, AHCA Notes. AHCA also publishes career training and educational materials relating to LTC.
Address: AHCA, 1201 L Street, NW, Washington, DC 20005-4014
Phone: (202) 842-4444; Fax: (202) 842-3860

American Health Security Act of 1993 (AHSA)

See also:
Corporate Alliance;
National Health Board (NHB);
Regional Health Alliance;
Universal Access (UNAC)

A proposal for national health care reform, submitted by President Clinton to Congress on October 27, 1993. The AHSA guarantees uninterrupted, comprehensive health coverage (i.e., *universal coverage*) for all Americans regardless of health or employment status. Coverage would be provided through a system of *regional* and *corporate health alliances*, which would pool the purchasing power of consumers and employers, thus stimulating health plans and providers to compete on the basis of quality, service, and price. An independent *National Health Board (NHB)* would set national standards and oversee the establishment and administration of the new health system by states. The NHB and existing government agencies would divide responsibilities for administration of the health care system at the national level. The Department of Health and Human Services would continue to administer existing programs, including Medicaid, Medicare, and Public Health Service. Financing would be through new taxes, individual and employer contributions, and Medicare and Medicaid savings.

American Hospital Association (AHA)

A national trade association representing nearly 5,500 hospitals, including general and specialized hospitals, corporate health care systems, and hospital-related providers of preacute and postacute services. AHA also has 16 personal membership groups and various associate memberships. The AHA represents members interests with legislators and government agencies, the media, and accrediting organizations (e.g., JCAHO) and develops policy positions and research. AHA publications, such as Hospitals & Health Networks, address current issues facing hospitals. Educational activities include national conferences, satellite teleconferences, and a resource center containing a collection of health care administration literature.
Address: AHA, 840 N. Lake Shore Drive,
Chicago, IL 60611
Phone: (312) 280-6000; Fax: (312) 280-3061

American Managed Care and Review Association (AMCRA)

A national trade organization representing approximately 500 managed care organizations (in 1993), including HMOs, PPOs, IPAs, UROs, HIOs, FMCs, and PROs. Membership also includes allied health professionals who provide services to the managed care industry. AMCRA provides educational programs, conducts research, promotes utilization review and quality assurance, communicates with legislative and governmental agencies, and serves as an information clearinghouse on legislative issues, industry trends, and statistics.
Address: AMCRA, 1227 25th St., NW, Suite 610,
Washington, DC 20037
Phone: (202) 728-0506; Fax: (202) 728-0609

American Medical Association (AMA)

See also:
Doctor of Osteopathy (D.O.);
Physician

The nation's largest professional organization for *physicians*, representing approximately 42% of the nation's 615,000 physicians in 1993. Membership is open to doctors of medicine (M.D.) and *doctors of osteopathy (D.O.)*. The AMA offers opportunities for education, professional development, and political advocacy. The AMA's proposal for health care reform calls for universal access to health care, malpractice reform, and controlled spending through market forces rather than mandatory caps on physicians' fees.
Address: AMA, 515 N. State Street,
Chicago, IL 60610
Phone: (312) 464-5000; Fax: (312) 464-5837

American Medical Peer Review Association (AMPRA)

See also:
Peer Review Organization (PRO)

A national trade association representing federally designated *peer review organizations (PRO)* under contract with the Medicare program. AMPRA's stated goal is to insure the incorporation of quality of care evaluation in national health care reform. AMPRA serves as the national policy voice for PROs, physician-directed medical review organizations, and individuals supportive of quality evaluation and improvement in peer review activities. The association works closely with various government agencies in developing regulations, budgets, and policies governing medical review programs in the public sector. Membership services include an information clearinghouse, educational seminars, national conferences, research on quality assessment tools and technology, and informational publications.
Address: AMPRA, 810 First St., NE, Suite 410,
Wahington, DC 20002
Phone: (202) 371-5610; Fax: (202) 371-8954

American Nurses Association (ANA)

See also:
Registered Nurse (RN)

A professional organization representing *registered nurses (RN)* through its 53 constituent associations, called State Nurses Associations (SNA). Through its SNAs, the ANA offers group purchasing advantages, develops nursing policy, lobbies for nursing and health care issues at the state and national levels, and presses for equitable salaries and working conditions. ANA also provides networking opportunities, research and educational events, legislative updates, publications, and certification programs through the American Nurses Credentialing Center (ANCC).
Address: ANA, 600 Maryland Ave., SW, Suite 100W, Washington, DC 20024-2571
Phone: (800) 274-4464; Fax: (202) 554-2262

American Society for Healthcare Risk Management (ASHRM)

See also:
American Hospital Association (AHA); Risk Management

A national professional society, organized as a component of the *American Hospital Association (AHA)*, representing professionals and students who are actively involved or otherwise interested in health care *risk management*. Members are hospital and other health care risk managers, nursing executives, administrators, commercial underwriters, insurance brokers, legal counsel, and consultants. The ASHRM provides its members a forum for the exchange of ideas and proven methodologies in health care risk management. Educational programs include annual conferences, workshops, seminars, research, publications, and other resources. ASHRM also monitors legislation affecting health care risk management and insurance.
Address: ASHRM, 840 N. Lake Shore Drive, Chicago, IL 60611
Phone: (312) 280-6430; Fax: (312) 280-4151

Americans with Disabilities Act (ADA)

A federal law enacted in 1992 which requires companies with 25 or more employees to take reasonable steps to accommodate disabled people already employed by the company as well as future hires. The ADA also states that a person's disabilities cannot be a factor in hiring or promoting unless those disabilities would prevent him/her from meeting the requirements of the job. Compliance with the law may require structural changes, purchases of special equipment, staff sensitivity training, re-defined job descriptions, or other changes that would enable the company to comply with the "spirit of the law." (In 1994, the ADA will apply to employers with 15 or more workers.)

Ancillary Services

See also:
Diagnostic Center

Supplemental medical services provided to patients to aid in the diagnosis and/or treatment of an illness or injury. Ancillary services may be diagnostic or therapeutic. They are rarely sought out by the patient without a referral by a physician. Examples of diagnostic ancillary services typically provided in a *diagnostic center* include: laboratory tests, radiology, electroencephalography (EEG), magnetic resonance imaging (MRI), ultrasound, echocardiology and other cardiac testing procedures. Examples of therapeutic ancillary services include: physical therapy, occupational therapy, speech therapy, and cardiac rehabilitation. Sometimes called *miscellaneous hospital charges.*

A

Anti-Kickback Statute

See: **Medicare/Medicaid Fraud and Abuse Statute**

Any Willing Provider

See also:
Closed Panel;
Preferred Provider

Refers to a law in some states mandating open participation in all managed care provider networks. An underlying purpose of this law is to preserve the patient's freedom of choice. For example, any provider that meets and accepts a managed care plan's parameters for participation cannot be excluded from the plan's *preferred provider* network. Most state laws allow for limited discrimination by PPOs if, for example, they want to exclude physicians with histories of poor medical care or hospitals that are geographically inconvenient. The "any willing provider" regulation directly impacts PPOs and managed care pharmacy networks, which attempt to control health care costs and quality by selectively contracting with providers who satisfy the quality requirements of the plan, monitoring their performance, and rewarding the most efficient providers. Managed care plans also rely on their ability to exclude certain providers as a competitive strategy.

Appeal

See also:
Expedited Appeal

A formal request to a claims processor, such as a utilization review organization (URO) or third party administrator (TPA), to reconsider a determination not to certify an admission, extension of stay, or other health care service.

Appropriate

See also:
Appropriate;
Appropriateness Review;
Medically Necessary

A determination by a claims processor, e.g., utilization review organization (URO) or third party administrator (TPA), during an *appropriateness review* that a medical service provided to a plan member is suited , that is, *appropriate* and *medically necessary*, for the presenting condition.

Appropriateness Review

See also:
Appropriate;
Medically Necessary;
Practice Guidelines

A utilization management technique used by third party payors in which individual cases are reviewed for clinical *appropriateness* and *medical necessity* of surgical and diagnostic procedures. The review usually consists of comparing clinical data to medical criteria. Because there is no single set of standards or review criteria universally used as management tools at this time, UROs often use different review criteria, require different information, and make considerably different decisions for similar kinds of clinical circumstances. However, physician *practice guidelines*, which are now being developed, may establish a common foundation for appropriateness review criteria.

Approved Charge

See also:
Customary, Prevailing, and Reasonable (CPR);
Fee Maximum (Fee Max)

The maximum fee that Medicare (or other managed care plan) will pay a provider in a given geographical area for a covered service.

Arbitration

See also:
Formal Grievance Procedure

The process by which the parties to a claims dispute submit their differences to the judgment of an impartial party appointed by mutual consent. Many managed care plans have compulsory arbitration provisions (in states where arbitration is allowed) covering disputes between plan members and providers in the plan's network. Arbitration is one of the last steps in the *formal grievance procedure* for resolving a plan member's complaint.

Assignment of Benefits (AOB)

A reimbursement method in which a claimant requests that his/her benefits under a claim be paid to some other designated person or institution (usually a physician or hospital). Assignment of benefits (AOB) eliminates the need for the patient to pay in full for services at the time they are rendered, then file a claim and await reimbursement from the health plan. Generally, the provider of care accepts the AOB as full payment for services rendered.

Authorization

See also:
Non-Participatory Provider (NonPar);
Out-of-Network Services (OON)

A utilization management technique used by HMOs whereby approval is given for care or services, such as hospitalization or evaluation by a physician specialist not on the HMO staff (i.e., *non-participatory provider*), for an HMO enrollee.

Average Daily Census (ADC)

See also:
Patient Day(s);
Weighted Daily Census (WDC)

The average number of hospital inpatients (other than newborns) per calendar day over a given period. The ADC is calculated as follows: the total number of *patient days* during a given period divided by the number of calendar days in that period.

Average Length of Stay (ALOS)

See also:
Admissions;
Bed Days;
Discharges;
Length of Stay (LOS)

The average number of days that the average patient remains in the hospital for a given time period. ALOS differs among various types of admissions. ALOS variations also exist by age and by sex. Generally, ALOS for a hospital is related to the unique case mix and practice style of its medical staff. The formula for calculating ALOS is: total number of *bed days* divided by the number of *admissions* or *discharges* during a specified period.

Average Payment Rate (APR)

See also:
Adjusted Average Per Capita Cost (AAPCC);
Adjusted Community Rate (ACR);
Medicare Risk Contract

The maximum amount of money that HCFA could pay an HMO or competitive medical plan (CMP) for services to Medicare beneficiaries under a *Medicare Risk contract*. The APR is calculated for a defined service area and then is adjusted for the enrollment characteristics that the plan would expect to have. The APR is derived from the *adjusted average per capita cost (AAPCC)*, which is the estimated cost of care for Medicare recipients under a cost-based Medicare arrangement for a given area. The actual payment to the HMO or CMP is the *adjusted community rate (ACR)*, which can never be higher than the APR.

Average Wholesale Price (AWP)

See also:
Blue Book

The standardized cost of a drug, which managed care plans frequently use for determining drug benefits. The AWP is determined through reference to a common source of price information, such as the American Druggist's *Blue Book*, which lists the costs charged for an undiscounted drug to a pharmacy by a large group of pharmaceutical wholesale suppliers. Wholesale costs are then averaged to yield the AWP.

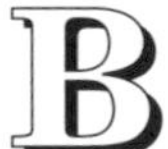

Balance Billing

See also:
No Balance Billing Clause;
Usual, Customary, and Reasonable (UCR)

The practice of billing the patient the difference between the provider's fee and the *usual, customary, and reasonable (UCR)* fee covered by the patient's insurance carrier.

Bed Days

See also:
Average Length of Stay (ALOS);
Length of Stay (LOS);
Patient Day(s)

A measurement of hospital utilization used by managed care plans to indicate the total number of days of hospital care (excluding the day of discharge) provided to a plan member in a given period. *Bed days* also may be used to measure outpatient surgery on the assumption that an outpatient surgical procedure will cost the plan about the same as a single inpatient day. *Bed days* usually is reported in "days per 1,000 plan members per year" and is used for calculating *average length of stay (ALOS).* Also called *hospital days, discharge days,* or *length of stay (LOS).* (Compare with *patient days.)*

Benchmarking

See also:
Best Practices;
Total Quality Management (TQM)

The process of searching for and implementing the *best practices* in the health care industry that lead to exceptional performance. Many providers are using benchmarking as a *total quality management (TQM)* technique for achieving organizational excellence. Benchmarking provides an organization an idea of where it stands in relation to competitors and a means for establishing goals within the organizational planning process. Benchmarking typically involves: 1) a continuous planning and strategy development process; 2) a search for creative solutions outside of the day-to-day environment; 3) a performance measurement process; and 4) a process of internal change.

Beneficiary

See also:
Eligible Person;
Member;
Recipient

Any individual who is eligible, as either a participant, subscriber, or dependent, for health care services provided under a health plan, as defined in the benefit(s) package. The term is frequently used in reference to Medicare participants.

Benefit Differentials

See also:
Out-of-Pocket Payments (OOP)

Refers to *out-of-pocket payments* (e.g., deductibles, coinsurance, and copayments) which the insured person is required to pay. In managed care plans, benefit differentials are structured so that benefits differ depending on whether covered services are received from preferred or non-participatory providers. For example, a plan may pay 80% of covered charges if the patient receives care from a provider in the plan's network. Thus, the plan has a 20% benefit differential. However, if the plan member receives care from a non-participatory provider, the plan may pay only 60% of covered charges, and the insured must pay the 40% benefit differential for the remainder.

Benefit(s) Package

See also:
Standard Benefits Package;
Certificate of Coverage (COC);
Covered Services

The combination of various medical services which a managed care plan or insurance carrier will cover for a plan member or policy holder. *Covered services* included in a benefits package are defined by the contract or insurance policy and are outlined in the *certificate of coverage (COC)* that is issued to the insured person.

Benefits

See also:
Benefit(s) Package;
Covered Services

Refers to the amount of money payable by a health plan for the cost of *covered services,* as defined in the *benefits package.*

Benefits Consultant

See also:
Employee Benefits Research Institute (EBRI); International Foundation of Employee Benefit Plans (IFEBP)

A person or company that specializes in the analysis and design of an employer's entire non-cash compensation package. Benefits consultants may also advise employers on employee benefits issues, such as legislation, cost-containment measures, marketplace trends, etc. As a continuing service to their clients, some benefits consulting firms act as third party administrators (TPA) of employee benefits plans. Benefits consultants are compensated directly by the employer, usually on a fee-for-service basis. Large, self-insured employers tend to use benefits consultants more than other employers. Also called *employee benefits consultant.*

Best Practices

See also:
Benchmarking; Total Quality Management (TQM)

Refers to organizations that have demonstrated superior performance in their clinical and operational processes, as indicated by formal comparative performance measures. Best practices may be identified by programs, such as *total quality management (TQM)*, which increase efficiency and productivity, improve quality, cut costs, increase revenues, market share and/or margins, or provide innovative operational approaches to service delivery. Best practices demonstrate not only highly successful clinical aspects of patient care but also management practices that contribute to their effectiveness. They also serve as *benchmarks* for other organizations that are trying to improve performance and quality. Providers with a "best practice" rating use it to their advantage in managed care contract negotiations.

Billed Charges

See also:
Fee-for-Service Reimbursement (FFS); Usual, Customary, and Reasonable (UCR)

A reimbursement arrangement whereby fees for health care services are based on what the provider usually charges all patients for the particular service. In other words, charges are billed on a "fee-for-service" basis. Billed charges generally are the most expensive reimbursement arrangement and are used mostly by traditional indemnity insurance companies. Also called *fee-for-service reimbursement (FFS).*

Birthing Center

A free-standing facility equipped to provide prenatal, delivery, and post-partum care for low risk pregnancies. Birthing Centers must meet all licensing requirements, which vary by state. For example, a state may require the Birthing Center to have at least one OB/Gyn physician specialist as its director, as well as nurses and staff who are trained for both normal delivery and medical emergencies. Birthing Centers also may be required to have ongoing quality assurance programs and a written agreement with a hospital in the area for emergency transfer of a patient or newborn. Generally, Birthing Centers provide services at a lower cost than hospitals.

Blanket Medical Expense

See also:
Maximum Allowable Payment (MAP)

An insurance policy provision that allows a covered person to collect up to the maximun amount of the policy for all hospital and medical expenses incurred without any limitations on individual types of medical expenses.

Blue Book

See also:
Average Wholesale Price (AWP);
Drug Price Review (DPR)

A pharmacy price schedule published by the American Druggist, which shows undiscounted costs of drugs charged by pharmaceutical wholesale suppliers. The Blue Book is used as a reference for a common source of price information and also for calculating the *average wholesale price (AWP)* of various drugs when managed care plans are determining drug benefits and price maximums during *drug price reviews (DPR).*

Blue Cross/Blue Shield Plans (BC/BS)

An umbrella term referring to 73 independent, non-profit, community-based Blue Cross and Blue Shield health plans, which together provide health care coverage to nearly 70 million Americans. Originally, Blue Cross and Blue Shield were organized as separate corporations, with Blue Cross providing protection against the cost of hospital services and Blue Shield covering the costs of physician office care. These distinctions, however, are no longer valid because many Blue Cross and Blue Shield plans have merged, though some remain separate depending on the plan and the state where they are operating.

Board Certified

See also:
Board Eligible; Certification

A term used to describe a physician who has completed a supervised program of certified clinical residency, passed examinations given by a medical specialty group, and, as a result, is certified as a specialist in his/her area of practice. Most hospitals and managed care plans require physicians on their staff and provider panels to be *board certified* or *board eligible.*

Board Eligible

See also:
Board Certified

A physician who is eligible to take a specialty board examination. *Board eligible* also includes those who may have failed the examination and remain eligible to take it again. To be board eligible, a physician must have graduated from a board-approved medical school, completed a period of supervised training, and practiced for a specified length of time. Government and other types of health programs that define standards for medical specialists often accept board eligibility as equivalent to board certification since the only difference is passing a specialty board examination.

Boarder Baby

A newborn that, for medical reasons, stays in the hospital longer than the normal healthy baby stay. (Typically, a normal, healthy newborn leaves the hospital when its mother is discharged). Sometimes called a *newborn boarder baby*.

Broker

See also:
Broker of Record

A person or independent agency who acts on behalf of employers in purchasing employee health care insurance. As a representative of the health care buyer, the broker solicits business and service contracts. However, unlike insurance company agents, brokers may place business with several insurers, though they may give one insurance carrier preference. Typically, brokers are paid a commission by the insurance company whose business they have placed with the employer. Commissions are usually based on a percentage of premium dues.

Broker of Record

See also:
Broker

A special designation given by an employer to a *broker*. The employer documents the broker of record status in a letter provided to the broker as written assignment of the broker's role with the employer. The letter identifies the broker as the only one that the insurance carriers are to pay a commission for placing the employer's insurance business until the letter is rescinded by the employer.

"Build or Rent"

See also:
Self-Funded Plan

A phrase commonly used in the employee benefits community to refer to an employer's decision whether to purchase a managed care program from a third party, such as an insurance carrier, or to develop and sponsor the program through the company itself (i.e., *self-funded plan)*.

Bundled Billing

See also:
Coronary Artery Bypass Graft Project (CABG); Global Fee

The practice of charging an all-inclusive package price, or *global fee*, for all medical services associated with selected procedures. HMOs and some specialty providers often use bundled billing for high-cost procedures (e,.g., organ transplants, heart surgery) and also for common procedures like maternity care, or for a year of care. A growing number of employers are negotiating bundled billing deals with providers in an attempt to control costs and improve quality of care. HCFA is experimenting with bundled billing in its Medicare "demonstration project" for *coronary artery bypass graft (CABG)* surgery. Also called a *global fee.*

Business Coalition

See also:
Direct Contracting; Health Care Coalition

An alliance of local employers in a community usually formed for the purpose of controlling health care costs without sacrificing quality or access to medical care. Business coalitions may serve as purchasing cooperatives for employees' health benefits. Many negotiate directly with hospitals on behalf of members, selectively choosing providers based on measures of quality, efficiency, and cost effectiveness. Business coalitions may be composed of large employers, small employers, or large and small employers together.

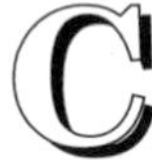

Cafeteria Plan

See also:
Flexible Benefit Plan (Flex Plan);
Section 125 Plan

A type of flexible employee health benefits program (*flex plan*) which permits employees to tailor coverage to meet their specific needs. Employees may select from among various cost, coverage and/or provider options. Flex plans which meet certain requirements under *Section 125* of the Internal Revenue Code may offer both taxable and non-taxable selections. Plans that do not wish to comply with IRS restrictions may offer choices among non-taxable benefits only. Also called *flexible benefit plan (Flex Plan).*

Calendar Year

See also:
Calendar Year Deductible

The period from January 1 of any year through December 31 of the same year, inclusive. The term is used in connection with deductibles (i.e., *calendar year deductible)* of major medical plans which provide benefits for expenses incurred within a calendar year.

Calendar Year Deductible

A deductible that applies to any covered medical expenses incurred by the insured during any one *calendar year.*

Call Schedule

See also:
After-Hours Care

A schedule that lists the physicians who are available for *after-hours care* for HMO enrollees. HMO physicians usually rotate on-call responsibilities since access to medical advice or care must be available 24 hours a day. In some staff model HMOs, a specialist is on call for all of the medical specialties in addition to a staffed after-hours care center.

Capitation (Cap)

See also:
Per Member Per Month (PMPM);
Risk Pool;
Risk Sharing

A type of *risk sharing* reimbursement method whereby providers in a plan's network receive fixed periodic payments (usually monthly) for health services rendered to plan members. Capitated fees are set by contract between a prepaid managed care plan (typically HMOs) and providers to be paid on a per person basis, usually with adjustments for age, sex, and family size, regardless of the amount of services rendered or costs incurred. The managed care plan may set aside a percentage of the total annual cap payment in a *risk pool* to safeguard against unexpected costs. At the end of the year, any money left in the risk pool is returned to the providers. *Capitation* can also refer to member enrollment fees. Within any given period (usually a year), the cost to the enrollee or to his/her employer for health benefits does not change regardless of the amount of services rendered. Capitation is usually expressed in units of *per member per month (PMPM).*

Carrier

Refers to an insurance company, a prepaid health plan, or a government agency that underwrites and/or administers a range of health benefits programs and any claims submitted by or for plan beneficiaries. In certain cases (e.g., HMOs), the carrier may provide health care services directly to enrollees.

Carryover

See also:
Calendar Year;
Deductible

A provision in many major medical plans that allows the covered person to avoid two *deductibles* when medical expenses are incurred in one *calendar year* and sickness or injury continues into the next year.

Carve-Out Service

See also:
Fee Schedule;
Specialty Network

A strategy used by some managed care plans to separately manage certain high-cost or specialty services, such as, mental health and substance abuse services, vision or dental benefits, etc. Carve-outs often save money for employers and also may provide more appropriate treatment for plan members. The aim is to manage care on an individual basis and make money available to pay for selected high-cost services that the patient needs, rather than tailoring treatment to available coverage. With respect to HMOs, carve-out services usually are certain normally covered services which may be subject to changing medical guidelines, for example, pharmacy benefits, mental health or chemical dependency benefits, and thus are excluded from coverage under standard HMO capitation payments. Such carve-out services may be reimbursed according to a *fee schedule*. Also called *clinical exclusions*.

C

Case Management

See also:
Case Manager (CM);
Utilization Management (UM)

A *utilization management* (UM) technique frequently used by third party payors and self-insured employers to monitor and coordinate treatment for specific diagnoses, particularly those involving high-cost or extensive services (e.g., mental health illnesses and chemical dependencies). The objective is to manage the costs and quality of high cost services. Case management may include case assessment, treatment planning, referral, and follow-up in order to ensure comprehensive and continuous service and coordinated payment and reimbursement. Also known as *large case management* or *catastrophic case management.*

Case Management Society of America (CMSA)

See also:
Case Manager (CM)

A professional society for *case managers (CM)* employed by managed care organizations, insurers, and case management companies and in independent practice. Membership benefits include educational and networking opportunities through annual conferences and educational forums. CMSA also represents members' interests in government affairs and legislative issues, and offers a Certification for Case Managers (CCM) credentialing program.
Address: CMSA, 1101 17th St., NW, Suite 1200, Washington, DC 20036
Phone: (202) 296-9200; Fax: (202) 296-0023

Case Manager (CM)

See also:
Case Management; Utilization Management (UM)

An experienced professional (usually a nurse, physician, or social worker) who handles catastrophic or high cost cases as a member of a *utilization management (UM)* team. Case managers (CM) work with patients, providers, and insurers to coordinate all health care services and resources in order to provide the patient with a plan of medically necessary and clinically appropriate health care. For example, CMs may prevent hospital admissions or initiate early discharges by coordinating alternative care services (e.g., home care, outpatient services). CMs also may negotiate discounts for various ancillary services, such as nursing care and pharmaceutical products.

Case Mix

See also:
Admissions/Admits

Refers to the relative frequency and intensity of hospital *admissions* for various diagnoses. Case mix reflects the different needs and uses of hospital resources and is used as a factor for determining the costs of services and for setting rates. Case mix can be based on different criteria, e.g., diagnosis, severity of illness, services utilization, or hospital characteristics.

Catastrophic Case Management

See: **Case Management**

Catastrophic Health Insurance

See also:
Major Medical Insurance;
Stop-Loss Reinsurance

A type of insurance beyond basic *major medical insurance* which covers severe or prolonged illnesses that may threaten financial ruin to an individual or family. Typically, a major medical plan will place a limit on claims and treatments of between $50,000 and $100,000. Anything that exceeds the limit is defined as "catastrophic" and is eligible for coverage under a catastrophic health insurance plan, if available. Usually catastrophic health plans have high benefit maximums, and also include some coinsurance.

Catchment Area

See also:
Catchment Area Management Project (CAM);
Civilian Health and Medical Program of the Uniformed Services (CHAMPUS);
Service Area

The geographical area from which a particular managed care plan or provider facility draws the bulk of its users. The catchment area may be delineated on the basis of population distribution, geographic boundaries, transportation accessibility, or other factors. For example, the Department of Defense defines a hospital's catchment area for its *CHAMPUS* demonstration project, called the *Catchment Area Management Project (CAM)*, as an area within a 40-mile radius surrounding the facility, specified by zip codes. Also called *service area*.

Catchment Area Management Project (CAM)

See also:
Catchment Area; Civilian Health and Medical Program of the Uniformed Services (CHAMPUS)

A managed care demonstration project within the federal government's *CHAMPUS* program in which alternative management techniques, such as a health care finder service, simplified claims processing, utilization management, and other modifications to the standard CHAMPUS benefits package, are used in an attempt to contain costs at the local level. In a CAM project, the military hospital commander is responsible for managing the delivery and financing of health care services for the entire CHAMPUS beneficiary population residing in a hospital's *catchment area* (a radius of approximately 40 miles). In 1992, five CAM demonstration projects were underway, each with unique operational features designed to take advantage of local geographical and health care environments.

Center of Excellence (COE)

See also:
Specialty Networks

A highly specialized product line or related product lines (e.g., neurosciences and orthopedics), selected by a provider for allocation of greater financial and management resources. Some providers develop centers of excellence (COE) as a strategy for differentiating themselves from competitors on the basis of quality of care. Others may develop COEs to increase their volume of admissions, enhance their reputation, or achieve greater economies of scale. COEs tend to deliver higher quality and more cost-effective care by virtue of the economies of scale achieved through higher patient volumes and more efficient use of resources. For these reasons, many managed care plans are incorporating COEs in their provider networks.

Certificate of Authority (COA)

See also:
State Health Planning and Development Agency (SHPDA)

Authorization issued by a state government for licensing the operation of an HMO within the state. Usually, COAs are issued by the *state health planning and development agency (SHPDA).*

Certificate of Coverage (COC)

A document provided to covered employees by the insurance carrier or managed care plan which outlines the benefits, covered services, and principle provisions of the group health plan provided under contract by the insurance carrier or managed care plan to the employer. COCs are required by state laws. Sometimes called *certificate of insurance (COI).*

Certificate of Insurance (COI)

See: **Certificate of Coverage (COC)**

C

Certificate of Need (CON)

See also:
State Health Planning and Development Agency (SHPDA)

A certificate issued in some states by a government oversight agency, such as the *state health planning and development agency (SHPDA),* to an individual or organization seeking permission to construct or modify a health facility, acquire major medical equipment, or offer a new or different health service. The purpose of the CON is to ensure that a facility or service will meet the needs of those for whom it is intended. Some states have dispensed with the CON requirement for certain types of health facilities and services. Federally qualified HMOs, however, are exempt from CON requirements in all states. Sometimes called *determination of need (DON).*

Certification

See also:
Accreditation;
Preadmission
Certification

A determination by a utilization review organization (URO) that an admission, extension of stay, or other health care service has been reviewed and, based on the information provided, meets the medical review requirements of a particular health plan. (See *preadmission certification.*)

Certification can also refer to a process by which either a government agency or a non-government association evaluates and recognizes (i.e., "certifies") a person who meets predetermined standards. Similar to the *accreditation* process for institutions.

Certified Nurse Midwife (CNM)

See also:
Allied Health
Professional;
Nurse Practitioner (NP)

A licensed *nurse practitioner (NP)* who is professionally trained in the care and delivery of obstetric patients and in neonatal care. Certified nurse midwives (CNM) usually work under the supervision of an obstetrician/ gynecologist (OB/GYN) and generally provide services at a lower cost than physicians. Managed care plans and providers in medically underserved areas where there are insufficient PCPs increasingly are using CNMs as a way to control costs and enhance the accessibility of maternity services.

CHAMPUS Reform Initiative (CRI)

See also:
Civilian Health and Medical Program of the Uniformed Services (CHAMPUS)

A government cost containment demonstration project designed to improve the quality and cost-effectiveness of the *CHAMPUS* program through competitive selection of "at risk" managed care contractors. The pilot program, started in 1988, offers two types of managed care products, an HMO, called CHAMPUS Prime, and a PPO, called CHAMPUS Extra. In addition to the typical utilization management techniques used by HMOs and PPOs, the CRI program also uses "health care finders." These are registered nurses (RNs) employed by CHAMPUS service centers who coordinate all patient referrals and resource sharing agreements between CRI contractors and military treatment facilities (MTF). CRI contractors provide staff, supplies, and equipment to the MTF in order to enhance patient care capability.

Charges

See also:
Fee Schedule

In managed care terminology, refers to the dollar amount owed to a participating provider for health care services rendered to a plan member, according to a *fee schedule* set by the managed care plan.

Chart Utilization Review

See also:
Utilization Management (UM);
Utilization Review (UR)

A type of *utilization review (UR)* procedure involving a retrospective analysis of individual medical records by trained health professionals for the purpose of assuring third party payors that appropriate and medically necessary care was provided to the plan member and properly billed. Chart utilization review is considered a powerful but time consuming and expensive *utilization management* tool for payors.

Chemical Dependency Services

See also:
Alcoholism Program;
Substance Abuse

Services and supplies used in the diagnosis and treatment of alcoholism, chemical dependency, and drug dependencies, as defined and classified by the U.S. Department of Health and Human Services (HHS).

Chemical Equivalents

See also:
Therapeutic Equivalents

Drug products that contain essentially identical amounts of the same active ingredients in equivalent dosage. Chemical equivalents usually are manufactured by different pharmaceutical companies and distributed by multiple vendors. Chemical equivalents must meet existing physical and/or chemical standards. Sometimes chemical equivalents are called *therapeutic equivalents,* though therapeutic equivalents are not necessarily chemically equivalent.

Chemotherapy

See also:
Oncology

A method of treatment for internal disease (usually cancer) involving the use of potent chemicals or drugs. Chemotherapy is designed to kill fast-growing microscopic cells, which generally include cancer cells as well as some normal cells, such as hair cells. Chemotherapy may be provided on an inpatient or outpatient basis. Inpatient costs usually are reimbursable by most health plans. Outpatient costs may or may not be reimbursable.

Chiropractor (D.C.)

See also:
Mandated Providers

A non-medical doctor who deals with the relationship of the nervous system and the spinal column in the restoration and maintenance of health. Doctors of Chiropractic (D.C.) must be licensed by a state board. In some states, coverage for chiropractic services are mandated benefits for group health plans, thus making D.C.s *mandated providers*.

Chronic Care

See also:
Acute Care

Treatment for a disease or health problem which manifests one or more of the following characteristics: 1) permanent; 2) leaves residual disability; 3) caused by nonreversible pathological alteration in health condition; 4) requires special training of the patient for rehabilitation; or 5) expected to require a long period of supervision, observation and care. The opposite of chronic care is *acute care.*

Churning

See also:
Medically Necessary

The practice by some providers of seeing a patient more often than is *medically necessary* primarily to generate more revenue through an increase in number of services provided. Churning, generally considered an unethical practice, usually is associated with performance-based reimbursement systems (e.g., fee-for-service), where there tends to be a heavy emphasis on productivity and providers are rewarded for seeing a high volume of patients.

Civilian Health and Medical Program of the Uniformed Services (CHAMPUS)

See also:
CHAMPUS Reform Initiative (CRI);
Military Health Services System (MHSS)

A federally funded program administered by the Department of Defense, which provides health care benefits delivered by civilian providers to retired U.S. military personnel and to dependents of active and retired members of the seven uniformed services of the U.S. The CHAMPUS program is part of the *Military Health Services System (MHSS).*

Claim

See also:
Assignment of Benefits (AOB);
Claimant;
Out-of-Network Services (OON)

An itemized statement of health care services and their costs provided by a hospital, physician's office, or other provider facility. Claims are submitted to the insurer or managed care plan by either the plan member (*claimant*) or the provider (see *assignment of benefits*) for payment of the costs incurred by the covered person. In most HMOs, the only time claims are submitted by enrollees is for reimbursement for care received from a non-HMO provider (see *out-of-network services*) on an emergency basis.

Claim Lag

See also:
Claim Lag Studies;
Date of Service

The length of time between the date on which a claim is incurred (i.e., the *date of service*) and the date on which the claim is paid.

Claim Lag Studies

See also:
Accrual;
Claim Lag

A claims management tool for tracking and tracing the length of time (i.e., "lag") between when a claim is incurred *(date of service)* and when it is paid. Claim lag studies are used to evaluate the reasonableness of managed care plans' advance estimates of medical expense claim *accruals*.

Claim Reserves

An amount of money set aside by an insurance carrier or prepaid health plan (i.e., HMO) in a reserve fund to ensure the fulfillment of financial commitments during a specified period (usually a policy year).

Claimant

See also:
Claim

A member of a health plan who files a *claim* for payment of benefits for covered services.

Claims Pooling

See also:
Community Rating;
Large Claim Pooling;
Physician Contingency Reserve (PCR);
Pooling

A technique in which claims are not charged exactly as they are experienced, but instead are "pooled" in order to obtain an average claims experience for the covered group. For example, in a *community-rated* health plan like an HMO, claims pooling is used to determine the premium for a group risk, based on the average claims experience of the plan's entire membership. Claims pooling also may be used to smooth the effects of random fluctuations in experience-based rating methods. Some prepaid health plans also use claims pooling for allocating claims to a physicians' risk-sharing fund, called *physician contingency reserve.*

Claims Review

See also:
Quality Assurance (QA);
Utilization Management (UM);
Utilization Review Organization (URO)

In claims processing, refers to the routine examination of a submitted claim in order to determine eligibility, coverage of services, and plan liability. Also refers to the review of unusual claims by a *utilization review organization (URO)* for items or services which fall into the gray area of claims processing (e.g., cosmetic surgery, experimental or investigational procedures). In these cases, claims review is part of the *quality assurance* and *utilization management* processes.

Clinic Without Walls (CWW)

See also:
Group Practice;
Multispecialty Group Practice (MSG)

A corporation formed by several physicans or some other party (e.g., hospital or managed care plan) for the purpose of managing the physicians' practices. Administrative and contracting functions are centralized even though the clinic without walls itself may be a geographically dispersed *multispecialty group practice (MSG).* All patient revenue is shared by the group. Reinsurance programs usually cover the risks that the doctors share with local hospitals. Typically, the CWW provides health care purchasers with fee schedules for specific procedures and episodes of care. A key advantage of a CWW is that physicians do not have to relocate their practices. They also retain autonomy over their office practices and compensation. In effect, the CWW arrangement creates a decentralized service delivery network which can enhance participating physicians' ability to contract with managed care plans. Sometimes called *group practice without walls (GPWW).*

Clinical Criteria

See also:
Preadmission Certification

The written policies, decision rules, medical protocols or guidelines used by a utilization review organization (URO) to determine *preadmission certification*, extension of stay, or other proposed health care service or treatment protocol for a plan member.

Clinical Exclusions

See: **Carve-Out Service**

Clinical Outliers

See also:
Diagnosis-Related Group (DRG)

Refers to atypical clinical cases that cannot be adequately assigned to an appropriate *diagnosis-related group (DRG)* because of unique combinations of diagnoses and surgeries, very rare conditions, or other unique clinical reasons.

Clinician

See also:
Practitioner;
Provider

A professionally trained hospital- or clinic-based staff member who provides technical medical services to patients. Usually this refers to physicians, but nurses may also be considered clinicians. Sometimes called a *practitioner or provider.*

Closed Panel

See also:
Group Model HMO;
Prepaid Group Practice Plan;
Staff Model HMO

A type of managed care plan that contracts with a limited selection, or "closed panel" of physicians on an exclusive basis. Closed panel plans usually require members to see a primary care physician who acts as a gatekeeper for care. Referrals to other providers must be only within the plan's closed panel of participating providers. This type of plan typically is found in *staff* and *group model HMOs*, but it also could apply to a large medical group practice that contracts with an HMO. In this case, the plan would be called a *prepaid group practice plan*. Also called *closed access*.

C

Coding

A classification method for identifying and defining physician services for billing and reimbursement purposes.

Coinsurance

See also:
Cost-Sharing Techniques;
First Dollar Coverage;
Out-of-Pocket Payments (OOP)

A form of cost-sharing whereby an insured individual pays a set percentage of the cost of covered medical services as an *out-of-pocket payment (OOP)* to the provider. A common coinsurance arrangement requires the insured to pay 20% of the cost of a health service and the plan pays the remaining 80%. Coinsurance differs from a *deductible* in that coinsurance provides *first dollar coverage*.

Collaboration

See also:
Horizontal Integration; Integrated Delivery System (IDS); Vertical Integration

A cooperative arrangement between two or more health care organizations for the purpose of better meeting community health care needs and reducing costs. As an alternative to competition, collaboration can eliminate overlap and duplication in the health care delivery system, reduce costs, improve access, enhance managed care contracting, or build a fully *integrated delivery system (IDS)*. Collaborative alliances may be set up among similar organizations (e.g., two hospitals, or several hospitals and a hospital system), or between different types of organizations, such as a hospital and a physician group or a hospital and a business coalition. Collaboration models range from relatively unstructured cooperative planning councils to formally structured legal entities, such as a for-profit joint development company, not-for-profit shared governance foundation, holding company, management service organization, merger, acquisition, consolidation, etc.

C

Combined Audit

See also:
Utilization Management (UM); Variation Analysis

A component of the *utilization management* process in which evaluation studies of patient medical care are conducted by an audit committee composed of physicians, nurses and/or professionals in other health care disciplines. Members of the audit committee jointly choose the same sample of records, utilize the same logic and the same data retrieval processes in their evaluations of patient care in order to ensure consistency and reliability. Criteria development and *variation analysis* may or may not be conducted separately for the medical care that is being audited.

Commercial Insurance

See also:
Fee-for-Service Insurance

Refers to traditional indemnity coverage (also known as *fee-for-service insurance)* provided by private or publicly owned for-profit insurance companies.

Commission

See also:
Administrative Costs

The portion of the insurance premium paid to a broker, insurance agent, or sales representative as compensation for services provided. Commissions usually are considered part of the *administrative costs* associated with the selling costs of a health plan.

Community Benefits

See also:
Voluntary Hospital

Activities initiated by not-for-profit providers (e.g., *voluntary hospitals*) to benefit the community in which the hospital operates. Community benefits are evolving standards defined by the Internal Revenue Service (IRS) for determining the tax-exempt status of not-for-profit health care organizations. Community benefits deemed "acceptable" by the IRS for tax-exempt status include: bringing a new service or provider to the community; sharing risk in a new activity; pooling diverse areas of expertise; improving patient convenience; increasing accessibility for patients; treating indigent patients; educational and research activites; increasing efficiency; reducing costs of care; enhancing quality of care and service. "Unacceptable" as community benefits, according to the IRS, are: soliciting patient referrals; improving one's financial status; and avoiding new competition.

Community Care Network (CCN)

See also:
American Hospital Association (AHA); Continuum of Care; Integrated Delivery System (IDS)

A local network of providers formed for the purpose of delivering comprehensive health services to an enrolled population within a community in return for predominantly capitated payments set by government agencies, or an independent regulatory body, or through marketplace negotiation. A CCN may be organized by an individual hospital, a group of hospitals, or other types of providers or non-provider entities (e.g., private insurers). Hospitals may own and operate the CCN, or have a partial equity interest in the network, or participate solely as a network member without equity interests and coordinating responsibilities. CCN is a term coined by the *American Hospital Association* to represent its concept of a restructured national health care system. The CCN concept emphasizes patient care management over cost management by organizing care delivery within a region or local community so that all needed services are efficiently provided and coordinated over time across providers, as a *continuum of care*.

Community Health Center (CHC)

See also:
Catchment Area; Community Oriented Primary Care (COPC)

A local, community-based ambulatory health care program organized and funded by the U.S. Public Health Service, which provides, either through its own staff or in conjunction with other resources, primary health services, preventive care, appropriate supplemental and environmental health services, and information on the availability of health services. CHCs usually serve a *catchment area* with scarce or non-existent health services, or a population with special health needs. CHCs often are called neighborhood health centers. However, the Health Revenue Sharing and Health Services Act of 1975 incorporated neighborhood health centers, family health centers, and community health networks under the single term *community health centers (CHC).* Similar non-federally funded community health programs, such as the *Community Oriented Primary Care (COPC)* program, may be sponsored by local hospital(s), public or private agencies, community foundations, managed care organizations, employers, business coalitions, etc.

Community Health Managed Information System (CHMIS)

See also:
Electronic Data Interchange (EDI); Management Information System (MIS)

A standardized, community-based, integrated computer system containing patients' health information on a computer network that links providers, payors, and state data banks. Patients who belong to a health plan that uses this type of information system carry a "smart card" (similar to a bank ATM card) containing patient demographics, medical conditions, and insurance information. CHMIS is expected to reduce administrative costs, speed up claims processing through electronic claims processing, improve the delivery of care within the community, and, ultimately, improve the health of community residents.

Community Oriented Primary Care (COPC)

See also:
Community Health Center (CHC)

A comprehensive, community-based integrated health care system designed to improve the health of medically underserved individuals who may not be able to access the health care system through conventional means. COPC provides easily accessible primary care, health maintenance, and medical intervention programs, based on a "one-stop shopping" concept whereby related services are located at one site. COPC programs attempt to reach uninsured people who do not typically seek treatment when their illnesses are still in early and more treatable stages. COPC also addresses social and cultural barriers that may exist for patients. The COPC approach first identifies the population considered at risk for a particular health problem, then develops a detailed plan to address that problem. Important components of the program are a system of financial incentives to staff members who meet stated goals and an emphasis on accountability, as measured by health outcomes. The COPC model was initiated in 1987 by Parkland Memorial Hospital in Dallas, TX, in cooperation with local universities, physicians, citizen groups, and a cooperative of existing clinics serving the poor.

Community Rating

See also:
Community Rating by Class (CRC); Experience Rating; Modified Community Rating

A rate-setting methodology in which capitation rates are determined without regard to characteristics of a subset of an enrolled population. For example, HMOs can vary premiums according to types of benefit packages. However, most state laws require HMOs to obtain the same amount of money per member for all members in the plan regardless of enrollees' health status. Thus, a group of enrollees that has characteristics likely to lead to higher utilization of health services cannot be charged a higher rate than a group expected to have low utilization of services.

Community Rating by Class (CRC)

See also:
Community Rating;
Industry Adjustment Factor (IAF);
Modified Community Rating

A variation of *community rating* in which prepaid health benefits rates may vary from group to group based on group differences in the proportions of enrolled persons in various demographic classes. Classes may be defined in terms of age, sex, family status, marital status, or other factors which may be used to predict expected differences in health risk for persons in the various classes. However, for all enrollees in a given class who have the same level of benefits and the same contract period, the rates are the same regardless of group affiliation or differences in the actual costs or use of services by enrollees within the class. The prepaid rates for a group reflect the community rates for each class, weighted by the number of that group's enrollees in each class. Sometimes called *modified community rating*.

C

Comorbidity

See also:
Outcomes Research;
Morbidity;
Severity -Adjusted Clinical Outcomes;
Severity of Illness Index

Refers to a medical condition that coexists with another diagnosed condition at the time of the patient's admission to a hospital and which increases the patient's *severity of illness*. Examples of comorbidities include: cancer, chronic cardiovascular disease, chronic liver disease, chronic renal disease, cerebrovascular degeneration, and diabetis melitus. Comorbidity measures are used in some clinical management information systems, such as the Acute Physiology and Chronic Health Evaluation (APACHE) system, for classifying admission severity and also in *outcomes research*. HCFA uses comorbidity as one of several measures to adjust for severity of illness at admission in order to predict mortality rates for Medicare patients and also to assess the effectiveness of care delivered to Medicare patients. Also called *substantial comorbidity*.

Competitive Medical Plan (CMP)

See also:
Medicare Risk Contract

A type of state-licensed health plan which delivers comprehensive, coordinated services to voluntarily enrolled members on a prepaid, capitated basis, similar to an HMO. CMP status may be granted by the federal government to a managed care plan, thus allowing the plan to obtain a *Medicare Risk contract* without having to qualify as an HMO. CMPs must meet specified criteria, but eligibility requirements are less restrictive than for an HMO.

Completed Audit

See also:
Combined Audit; Variation Report

The written report of a patient's medical care evaluation study (*combined audit*) in which variation records have been analyzed and corrective actions formulated for any problems identified. The audit procedure is not considered complete until follow-up of the problem has been planned and final reports (e.g., *variation report*) have been forwarded to pertinent medical and professional staff as well as the hospital's governing body.

Compliance

See also:
Non-Compliance

Refers to a patient's cooperation in voluntarily following the written instructions for using a drug or other prescribed treatment regimen. In order to reduce the risk of *non-compliance*, some drug manufacturers are developing innovative uses of information technology. For example, a microprocessor placed inside the cap of a drug container can beep to remind patients when to take their medication. The device also can record when and how much of the drug is taken. This information then can be downloaded to a PC computer for review by a physician, pharmacist or managed care company.

Complication

See also:
Iatrogenic Disease

An unanticipated change in a patient's clinical status during a hospital stay which may prolong the length of stay. Complications also can occur in ambulatory patients. The complication may require special clinical management to achieve desired outcomes.

Composite Rate

A group billing rate which applies to all plan members within a given group, regardless of whether they are enrolled for single or family coverage.

Comprehensive Major Medical Insurance

See also:
Catastrophic Health Insurance; Corridor Deductible; Major Medical Insurance

A type of health plan which combines basic and major medical coverages in a single plan. Comprehensive major medical insurance usually has a low deductible (e.g., $100) and a high maximum benefit. Typically, most medical expenses are covered under this type of plan. For example, after the initial deductible, the plan might pay 100% of hospital expenses up to a certain limit, after which the plan would pay a percentage (e.g., 80%) of all other expenses, including hospital expenses that exceed the limit.

Computerized Axial Tomography (CAT)

See also:
Ancillary Services; Diagnostic Center

A diagnostic radiological imaging procedure which uses a minicomputer and highly sensitive X-Ray detectors to produce extremely accurate three dimensional images of body and brain tissue. CAT is considered an *ancillary service* which often is provided in an outpatient *diagnostic center*.

Concurrent Review

See also:
Utilization Management (UM);
Utilization Review (UR)

A *utilization management* technique used by managed care organizations to ensure that medically necessary and appropriate care is delivered during a plan member's hospitalization episode. Concurrent reviews are conducted by trained health care professionals via telephone or on-site visits during plan members' hospital stays. Typically, reviewers monitor the course of routine medical procedures, as well as length of stay and discharge planning. Sometimes called *on-site concurrent review (OSCR).*

Consolidated Omnibus Budget Reconciliation Act of 1985 (COBRA)

See also:
Continuation of Coverage

A federal law which, among other things, requires employers to offer employees and their dependents who would otherwise lose their group health plan eligibility (typically, due to termination of employment) *continuation of coverage* under the firm's group plan. Employers are required to make health plans available for periods ranging from 18 to 36 months. COBRA legislation specifies rates, coverage, qualifying events, eligible individuals, notification requirements and payment terms. Another part of the COBRA legislation relates to Medicare beneficiaries in that it makes it easier for them to disenroll from a Medicare Risk contract with an HMO or CMP.

Consumer Price Index (CPI)

See also:
Producer Price Index-Hospital (PPI-H)

An economic barometer used by the Department of Labor's Bureau of Labor Statistics to measure national price changes over time. CPI measures the average change in retail prices paid by consumers for various goods and services. CPI also has medical and hospital components, called the *Consumer Price Index Medical Care Services (CPIMCS)* component. The CPI-MCS measures only out-of-pocket health care expenditures by consumers and does not include expenditures from any other sources, such as Medicare and Medicaid. Some observers believe that the CPI-MCS is a poor indicator of national health prices because it may overestimate the rate of general medical care price increases, since most health care services are purchased by third parties (insurers, managed care plans, government programs), who pay significantly lower, discounted price. In addition to the MCS component, CPI has a pharmaceutical component, called the CPI-Rx, which reflects the retail prices of drug products by type.

Consumer Price Index-Medical Care Services (CPI-MCS)

See: **Consumer Price Index (CPI)**

Continuation of Coverage

See also:
COBRA

A situation where an insured person who would otherwise lose coverage under a health plan due to certain occurrences, such as termination of employment or divorce, is allowed to continue his/her coverage under specified conditions and length of time (generally, 18 to 36 months). Continuation of coverage is a requirement specified in the *COBRA* legislation.

Continued Stay Review (CSR)

See also:
Utilization Review (UR)

A utilization review committee's review and initial determination during a plan member's hospitalization of the medical necessity and appropriateness of continuation of the patient's stay at a hospital at a particular level of care. Also called *recertification*.

Continuing Care Retirement Community Program (CCRC)

See also:
Life Care at Home Program (LCAH); Long-Term Care (LTC)

A type of *long-term care (LTC)* program for Medicaid patients which combines the financing and delivery of long-term care coverage within a single organizational context and insures residents against the catastrophic costs of long-term care. CCRCs offer housing and related services, and often include medical, preventive health and nursing home care. Most CCRCs provide plan members with some level of nursing home insurance. Some provide nursing care on a strictly fee-for-service basis. (Compare with a *life care at home program.*)

Continuity of Care

See also:
Continuum of Care; Integrated Delivery System (IDS)

Broad-based health care which provides medical services on a coherent and continuing basis, beginning with a plan member's initial contact with a provider through all episodes of the patient's medical care needs (i.e., from "cradle to grave"). Also called a *continuum of care.*

Continuous Quality Improvement (CQI)

See also:
Quality Assurance (QA); Quality Improvement Program (QIP); Total Quality Management (TQM)

A key component of a *total quality management (TQM)* program which involves rigorous, systematic, organization-wide processes to achieve ongoing improvement in the quality of products, services and operations, and the elimination of waste. Many health care organizations are embracing CQI programs as a way to improve quality, and also as a strategy for differentiating services from their competitors' services. Unlike traditional *quality assurance* programs, CQI programs focus on both outcome and process of care. CQI assumes that problems are the result of defects in the larger structure or system within which the individual functions rather than human error. Also called *quality improvement program (QIP).*

Continuum of Care

See also:
Continuity of Care; Integrated Delivery Systems (IDS)

The full range of services for all aspects of health care, including prevention, wellness, primary care, specialty care, acute care, sub-acute care, nursing home, hospice and home care, for patients in a defined geographic area. The services may include: public health education, immunizations, wellness programs, ambulatory care clinics, outpatient diagnostic and laboratory services, acute care, tertiary care services, rehabilitation, psychiatric care, long-term care, congregate living, and hospice care. A continuum of care is a key characteristic of *integrated delivery systems (IDS).*

Contract Compliance Audit

A contract management technique used by providers to ensure that payments received from third party payors are correct. Contract compliance audits also can uncover areas of problem payments as well as identify required changes to existing contracts, often resulting in increased revenue.

Contributory Plan

See also:
Evidence of Insurability (E of I); Medical Expense Reimbursement Plan (MERP); Non-Contributory Plan

A type of employer-sponsored group health plan under which employees share in the cost of the plan by paying a portion of the premium, usually through payroll deductions. Eligible employees normally have 30 days to enroll in a contributory plan without having to submit medical *evidence of insurability (E of I).* This is called the enrollment period. If employees (or their dependents) do not enroll during this period, they still may enroll later, but coverage will be subject to medical evidence of insurability, such as medical review, physician statement, etc. By contrast, in a *non-contributory plan,* or *medical expense reimbursement plan (MERP)*, the employer pays the entire cost of the plan, including out-of-pocket expenses. Enrollment periods do not apply to non-contributory plans because they require 100% employee participation.

Conversion Factors

See also:
Physician's Current Procedural Terminology, 4th Edition (CPT-4) Relative Value Scale (RVS)

The dollar amounts used in calculations for estimating the average cost per service for physician services. Conversion factors are multiplied by *relative value scale (RVS)* units, which vary by medical procedure according to the relative complexity (i.e., cost) of the different procedures, as coded by *CPT-4 Physician Procedure Codes*. Conversion factors vary by geographical area and time period. They are used by managed care plans to estimate prevailing physician fee levels for a given community and calendar year.

Conversion Plan

See also:
Continuation of Coverage

A type of group health plan which allows plan members to change their coverage to an individual policy without providing evidence of insurability. The conditions for conversion are defined in the group contract. Typically, a conversion is made when a covered person leaves the group, for example, at termination of employment. Conversion to an individual policy, however, may result in different benefits and rates.

Coordinated Care

See also:
Alternative Delivery System (ADS); Coordinated Care Program (CCP); Managed Care; Managed Competition

An alternative term for *managed care* or *alternative delivery systems (ADS)* coined during the Bush administration by HCFA's Office of Coordinated Care Policy and Planning (OCCPP). Coordinated care refers to standard managed care programs (e.g., HMOs, PPO, EPOs, POS), as well as indemnity plans that incorporate managed care techniques, like utilization management and discounted fees, and other cost- control techniques used by many employers, such as self-insuring, reducing covered benefits, and increasing employee cost-sharing. Since President Clinton took office, the term is used infrequently, having been replaced by the term *managed competition* to describe the model favored by the Clinton administration for a reformed national health care system.

Coordinated Care Program (CCP)

See also:
CHAMPUS;
Coordinated Care;
Military Health Services System (MHSS)

A health care reform initiative of the *Military Health Services System (MHSS)* designed to provide commanders of military treatment facilities the tools, authority, and flexibility to improve access to health care services, control costs, and ensure quality care to all MHSS beneficiaries. The Coordinated Care Program (CCP) begun in 1992, is being phased in over a three-year period. The CCP attempts to coordinate direct military care and indirect civilian health care sytems (e.g., *CHAMPUS*). Key features of the program include: an open enrollment system, cost-sharing incentives, a system of primary care managers and health care networks, and improved utilization management and quality assurance programs.

Coordination of Benefits (COB)

See also:
Duplicate Coverage Inquiry;
Duplication of Benefits;
Primary Payer;
Secondary Coverage

A cost-control mechanism used by most insurance companies to prevent a covered person from receiving duplicate benefits, that is, payments for medical services from two or more insurers. When an individual has duplicate coverage (see *duplication of benefits*) from two or more insurance carriers, coordination of benefits (COB) determines which carrier is the *primary payer* and must pay up to the limit of its policy. The other insurer then is designated the secondary payer and must pay any remaining amount covered by the plan. The purpose of COB is to ensure that no person or entity is reimbursed for more than the total cost of the care or services provided.

Copayment (CoPay)

See also:
Cost-Sharing Techniques; Out-of-Pocket Payments (OOP)

A *cost-sharing technique* whereby a plan member or insured individual pays a specified amount of money directly to a provider out of his/her own pocket (*out-of-pocket payment)* at the time services are rendered. The managed care plan or insurance carrier pays the remaining amount. Usually the copayment is a fixed amount, such as $5.00 per visit in many HMOs. Copayments are intended to control utilization.

Core Coverage

See also:
Non-Core Coverage

Refers to basic medical benefits which usually exclude dental and vision benefits.

Coronary Artery Bypass Graft Project (CABG)

See also:
Bundled Billing; Simplified Payment Method

A three-year experimental Medicare project (started in June, 1991) underway at selected hospitals. The project's goals are to: 1) test the feasibility of using an all-inclusive payment (i.e., *bundled billing)* for hospital and physician services associated with coronary artery bypass graft (CABG) surgery; 2) determine if Medicare beneficiaries can be encouraged to receive care at selected centers; and 3) monitor, measure, and report on clinical outcomes associated with CABG surgery. The project uses a *simplified payment method* in which all costs associated with the CABG procedure are bundled together. Medicare pays a lump sum per bypass case, ranging from $21,092 to $35,182, depending on the hospital and complexity of the procedure. Hospitals may seek small additional payments from insurers that provide supplemental coverage. However, participating hospitals and physicians agree not to bill patients separately. Patients are still responsible for any deductibles and coinsurance. *Note: The acronym CABG refers to both the surgical bypass procedure and the Medicare demonstration project related to the procedure.*

Coronary Care Unit (CCU)

See also:
Intensive Care Unit (ICU)

A specialized unit in a hospital designed to treat patients with serious cardiac diseases using specialized equipment and staff to provide continual patient monitoring.

Corporate Alliance

See also:
American Healthcare Security Act (AHSA); Regional Health Alliance

Under President Clinton's health care reform proposal, called the *American Healthcare Security Act* (AHSA), companies with more than 5,000 employees would be allowed to form their own "corporate alliance" rather than join a *regional health alliance.* The corporate alliance would be required to provide the same federally guaranteed benefits package and meet virtually all other government guidelines for alliances. It could provide health benefits to eligible employees, either through a certified self-funded employee benefit plan or through contracts with state-certified health plans. Corporate alliances would be governed by the Department of Labor. If the number of employees at a company falls below 4,800, the employer would be required to join the regional health alliance. Once an employer joins a regional alliance, it would not have the option to form a corporate alliance later on.

Corridor Deductible

See also:
Integrated Deductible

A special deductible which separates a basic medical plan from a supplementary major medical plan. The corridor deductible represents the portion of covered expenses that must be paid by the covered person before the major medical plan provides benefits. Also called *integrated deductible.*

Cosmetic Treatment

See also:
Elective Surgery; Medically Necessary

Services provided by physicians or dentists that are not deemed *medically necessary* and often involve elective surgery aimed at improving appearance. Generally, cosmetic treatments are not covered under most health plans. However, cosmetic surgery for prompt repair of accidental injury or for the improvement of the functioning of a malformed body part usually is covered by health plans. In such cases, the procedure is usually referred to as *reconstructive surgery.*

Cost-Based Reimbursement

See also:
Fee-for-Service Reimbursement (FFS); Retrospective Reimbursement

A method of paying providers for actual costs incurred by plan members. Generally, the costs for health care services must conform to explicit principles defined by third party payors. Sometimes called *retrospective reimbursement* or *fee-for-service reimbursement (FFS).*

Cost-Sharing Techniques

See also:
Contributory Plans; Cost-Shifting; Out-of-Pocket Payments (OOP)

Various strategies which many employers use to reduce employee health benefits costs by requiring employees to pay a portion of the health care costs. Deductibles, coinsurance, copayments, employee contributions for premiums, and benefit limitations are examples of common cost-sharing techniques. They frequently are used in *contributory plans* to reduce use of health care services, since employees must contribute out of their own pockets toward a portion of their own health care. Sometimes cost-sharing is called *cost-shifting*, though this is not entirely accurate. Cost-shifting has a broader meaning which applies to a wide variety of tactics used by the federal government, hospitals, physicians, managed care plans, large and small employers, insurance carriers, and other health care stakeholders to contain their own costs at the expense of other stakeholders.

Cost-Shifting

See also:
Cost-Sharing Techniques

A term used to describe how one patient's health care is subsidized by higher charges to another patient for the same services. For example, a provider redistributes the dollar difference between normal charges and reimbursement from certain payors (typically, payors with capitated or discounted payment agreements, also charity care) by increasing charges to other payors (usually fee-for-service payors). Medicare and Medicaid are leaading causes of cost-shifting. By limiting payments for services to beneficiaries, these government programs compel providers to collect the difference from other patients. Cost-shifting also occurs when managed care plans use their negotiating leverage to control provider expenses. As a result, providers shift their costs to fee-for-service plans, forcing these plans to raise premiums to offset losses.

Counterdetailing

See also:
Generic Substitution Program; Therapeutic Equivalents

A cost-control practice whereby drug therapy experts, typically employed by insurers and managed care plans, inform drug prescribers, either face-to-face or by letter or telephone, about the cost benefits of related kinds of drug therapy. Counterdetailers particularly stress the use of *generic substitutes* and *therapeutic equivalents* which usually are less costly than branded drugs. Drug manufacturers traditionally have used drug salespeople, known as "detailers," to inform physicians of new drug products and provide prescribers with free samples. The advent of counterdetailing, with its emphasis on cost-effectiveness, is forcing many drug companies to alter their traditional detailer-based sales strategy to accommodate the interests of managed care buyers.

Coverage

See also:
Benefit(s) Package; Covered Services

Health care benefits, or *covered services*, provided to eligible persons under a health benefit plan.

Covered Expenses

See also:
Coverage; Major Medical Insurance

Hospital, medical and miscellaneous health care expenses incurred by an insured person which entitle him/her to a payment of benefits under the terms of a health plan. The term is used mostly in connection with *major medical insurance* coverage in which "covered expenses" defines the type and amount of expense that is considered in the calculation of benefits.

Covered Person

See also:
Eligibility; Eligible Person

An *eligible person* who meets a health plan's *eligibility* requirements and for whom premium payments are paid for specified benefits of the contract between an insurance carrier and a contract holder.

Covered Services

See also:
Benefit(s) Package; Eligible Expenses

Specific health care services and products for which reimbursement is provided under the terms of the group health plan.

Credentialing

See also:
Staff Privileges

A process of checking a practitioner's references and documentating his/her credentials, including training, experience, demonstrated ability, licensure verification, malpractice insurance, etc. Credentialing is carried out by both hospitals and managed care organizations to ensure that only qualified practitioners with current, demonstrated competence have practice privileges at the hospital or other type of health care facility,and that they practice within the range of their expertise and abiliites. Often, managed care organizations defer to hospitals for credentialing of physicians and non-physician staff. Some plans, however, establish their own credentialing programs. Hospitals and managed care organizations both may be held liable for corporate negligence in their selection of practitioners who do not meet credentialing criteria for clinical *staff privileges*.

Cumulative Trauma Disorder (CTD)

See also:
Ergonomic Hazard; Occupational Disease

A work-related disorder which develops over time as a result of worker exposure to *ergonomic hazards*. For example, a worker who performs repetitive and/or prolonged wrist motions might develop pain and numbness in the hand and wrist, which results in a reduction in his/her productivity. CTDs account for an increasingly large percentage of workers' compensation costs each year, and represent nearly half of the *occupational diseases* reported in the annual Bureau of Labor Statistics (BLS) survey.

Current Procedural Terminology (CPT)

See also:
Physician's Current Procedural Terminology, 4th Edition (CPT-4)

A classification system of terminology and coding developed by the American Medical Association and used for describing, coding, and reporting medical services and procedures. Also known as *Physician's Current Procedural Terminology, 4th Edition (CPT-4).*

Custodial Care

See also:
Activities of Daily Living (ADL)

Patient care that is not medically required but is necessary when the patient is unable to care for himself/herself. Custodial care may involve medical or non-medical services which do not seek to cure, but are provided during periods when the patient's medical condition is not changing. Custodial care services, such as assistance in the *activities of daily living (ADL),* normally do not require ongoing administration by medical personnel. This type of care usually is not covered under managed care plans. Also called *domiciliary care.*

Customary Charge

See also:
Approved Charge;
Customary, Prevailing, and Reasonable (CPR);
Supplier;
Usual, Customary, and Reasonable (UCR)

The usual charge by a physician, hospital, or *supplier* for particular services or products. Customary charge also refers to the maximum amount that a Medicare carrier or other payor will approve for payment for a particular service by a provider, barring special circumstances. This maximum, or *approved charge*, is based on data of actual charges for a specific service performed by one provider for all of its patients.

Customary, Prevailing, and Reasonable (CPR)

See also:
Approved Charge; Customary Charge; Medicare Economic Index (MEI)

Medicare's method for determining the *approved charge* for a particular Medicare Part B service from a specific physician or supplier. In the CPR method, the approved charge is the lowest of the following three charges: the physician's actual charge for the service, the physician's *customary charge* for the service, and charges made by peer physicians or suppliers in the same geographical area. Prevailing charges are adjusted, if necessary, by the *medicare economic index (MEI).*

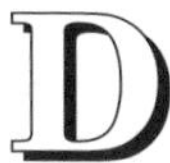

Data Retrieval

See also:
Utilization Review (UR)

The process of gathering patient care data from medical records for *utilization review.* The retrieved patient data usually is presented on a "data retrieval and analysis" form, which shows the details of compliance or non-compliance with review criteria and the audit committee's decision regarding instances of non-compliance with criteria.

Date of Service (DOS)

In claims processing, the date on which health care services were provided to the covered person.

Day Surgery

See also:
Ambulatory Care; Free-Standing Outpatient Surgery Center

Refers to intermediate level surgical procedures that usually are too complex to be performed in a physician's office but do not require inpatient hospitalization. Typically, day surgery requires shorter recovery periods (generally less than 24 hours) and is less costly than inpatient surgery. Day surgery may be performed at *free-standing outpatient surgery centers, surgi-centers,* and hospital-based outpatient surgery centers. Also called *outpatient* or *ambulatory surgery.*

Deductible

See also:
Copayment (CoPay);
Cost-Sharing Techniques

The portion of health care expenses which a plan member or insured person must pay "out-of-pocket" before any insurance coverage applies or reimbursement for expenses begins. Deductibles are usually tied to some time period over which they must be incurred, such as per calendar year, per benefit period, or per episode of illness. Use of deductibles is a *cost-sharing technique* commonly used by insurance plans and PPOs. Their purpose is to encourage utilization of services only when necessary and also to discourage submission of small claims due to the administrative expense involved in claims processing. Deductibles are not allowed in federally qualified HMOs and usually are not permitted under state HMO regulations. However, HMO *copayment* requirements can achieve the same result.

Deductible Carryover Credit

See also:
Calendar Year Deductible;
Carryover

Charges applied to the *calendar year deductible* for health care services provided during the last few months of a calendar year which may be used to partially or fully satisfy the following year's deductible. Deductible carryover credit may be used even if the deductible for the prior calendar year has not been met.

"Deep Pocket"

Refers to a hospital (usually) or other health care organization that is sued along with other defendents primarily because the organization is perceived as a greater source of settlement funds than other defendents, even though the organization may be involved in the case only by association.

Defensive Medicine

See also:
Malpractice;
Malpractice Insurance

Refers to changes in clinical practice patterns often involving medically unnecessary tests and procedures carried out by health care providers for the sole purpose of avoiding *malpractice* litigation. Defensive medicine may include *positive* defensive activities (found most often in high-risk physician specialties), such as diagnostic tests, performance of additional procedures, calling in consultants or sub-specialists, more follow-up tests, etc., and *negative* defensive activities, such as restricting practice to low-risk patients, ceasing to perform high-risk procedures, and retiring from practice because of liability concerns.

Deferred Premium Plan

See also:
Claim Reserves

A type of group health plan funding arrangement in which the employer is allowed up to sixty or ninety days to pay the current month's premium. This enables the employer to retain funds for investment income instead of paying out the funds to the insurer. Ordinarily, conventionally funded plans allow the employer a thirty-one day grace period during which the premium for the current month is overdue but payable without allowing the policy to lapse. Deferred premium plans are the simplest of all alternative health plan funding arrangements. Since ninety days' worth of premium is roughly equivalent to the reserves required by the insurance carrier, the deferred premium arrangement effectively eliminates the cash *claim reserves* usually held by the insurer.

D

Deficiency Analysis

See also:
Utilization Review (UR)

A review of any medical records that did not pass audit committee's *utilization review* in order to assess the extent of clinical problems and plan corrective measures to recommend.

Delete

See also:
Accrete

A term used by HCFA to describe the process of removing an individual from a health plan's Medicare program. The antonym is *accrete*.

Demand

The amount of a given health care service sought by consumers in response to their perceived need for that service.

Demographics

See also:
Psychographics

The study of the characteristics of a given population. Examples of demographic data include birth rate, age and sex composition, urban/rural distribution, mobility, income, household types, etc. Demographics are useful for strategic planning, product analysis, marketing and market management.

Dental Maintenance Organization (DMO)

See also:
Closed Panel

A type of managed dental care plan which provides comprehensive dental services to enrollees for a fixed per capita fee, similar to an HMO. Generally, in a DMO dental services are provided by a *closed panel* of dentists.

Dental Service Corporation

A not-for-profit organization that underwrites and/or administers contracts for managed dental care plans.

Dependent

See also:
Eligible Person

An individual other than a health plan subscriber who is eligible (i.e., meets the requirements specified in the group contract to qualify for coverage) to receive health care services under the subscriber's contract. Generally, dependents are limited to the subscriber's spouse and minor children. Premium payments are usually higher for dependent coverage than for individual coverage.

Detoxification

See also:
Alcoholism Program;
Substance Abuse

Refers to medical management of a patient's care while the individual withdraws from alcohol or other chemical or drug dependency.

Diagnosis

See also:
Principal Diagnosis

Identification or determination of the nature of a disease or condition through analysis and examination of its signs and symptoms.

Diagnosis-Related Group (DRG)

See also:
DRG Payment Method; Medicare

An inpatient classification system used by HCFA to determine hospital reimbursement for Medicare patients. The Diagnosis-Related Group (DRG) system categorizes patients with similar medical diagnoses, treatment patterns, and statistically comparable lengths of stay in a hospital. HCFA pays the hospital a fixed rate, based on the average expected use of hospital resources for each DRG in a given geographical area. The national DRG-based reimbursement system for Medicare patients began in late 1983. Some managed care plans and insurers are now adopting the *DRG payment method* for setting their payment rates and selecting providers.

Diagnostic Center

See also:
Ancillary Services

A facility, either free-standing or hospital-based, which specializes in the diagnosis of illnesses and injuries. Diagnostic centers typically have sophisticated diagnostic equipment for performing complex technological procedures, such as magnetic resonance imaging (MRI), computer assisted tomography (CAT), and ultrasound.

Direct Contracting

See also:
Discounted Charges; Exclusive Provider Organization (EPO)

Refers to an exclusive contractual arrangement between an employer and a hospital, or other provider organization, for health care services, usually provided at reduced prices for employee groups. The two parties may negotiate charges for services in a variety of ways, such as *discounted charges*, per diem rates, or billings based on anticipated revenues, admissions, or DRGs. Direct contracts may include use of third party administrators for processing claims and performing utilization management. Frequently, employers use direct contracting as a cost containment strategy. Providers generally use a direct contracting strategy to increase market share.

Direct Payment Subscriber

A person enrolled in a prepaid health plan who makes individual premium payments directly to the plan rather than through a group. Rates are generally higher for direct payment subscribers. Also, benefits may not be as extensive for the direct payment subscriber as for a subscriber enrolled and paying as a member of a group plan. Sometimes called *non-group subscribers*.

Disbursed Self-Funded Plan

See also:
Self-Funded Plan; Stop-Loss Reinsurance

A type of *self-funded plan* in which employees' claims are paid directly out of the employer's cash flow as part of the expense of doing business. In other words, the employer does not set aside claim reserves, nor does it pay premiums to an insurer. Claims settlements are tax deductible when they are paid rather than when they are incurred. Since a self-funding company assumes all the financial risk, most companies that use a disbursed self-funded plan also buy stop-loss insurance in order to protect themselves against significantly poorer-than-expected experience.

Discharge Days

See: **Bed Days** and **Length of Stay (LOS)**

Discharge Planning

See also:
Aftercare

A centralized, coordinated hospital program in which a trained health care professional identifies and evaluates the anticipated health care needs of a patient following his/her discharge from the hospital. Discharge planners also arrange for appropriate *aftercare*. Managed care organizations often coordinate their own discharge planning processes with hospital discharge planners in order to provide health plan coverage information and also to assist in acquiring necessary services or equipment for the patient to survive in a non-hospital environment.

Discharge Status

See also:
Against Medical Advice

Refers to the disposition of the patient upon discharge or release from a medical facility. For example, the patient who returns home after hospitalization has a discharge status of "home." The patient who leaves the hospital without the permission of his/her physician or the knowledge of hospital personnel is given a discharge status of *against medical advice.*

Discharges

See also:
Admissions

Refers to the number of patients who leave (i.e. are discharged from) an overnight medical care facility (usually a hospital, but sometimes an extended care facility) in a given time period. The antonym is *admissions*.

Discounted Charges

See also:
Billed Charges;
Risk Sharing

A common *risk sharing* method of managed care reimbursement, whereby a provider agrees to reduce its *billed charges* for services by some percentage in exchange for a significant and/or predictable amount of business from a managed care plan. Often, the basis for a fee schedule is a discount off of prevailing fee levels, which typically vary by region and other factors. The discounted charges reimbursement method has some risks for providers. For example, some managed care plans try to negotiate 10% to 20% discounts off billed charges. If the discounted payment doesn't cover the provider's fixed costs, the provider loses money. Any incremental business delivered by the managed care plan then magnifies those losses.

Discounted Fee-for-Service

See also:
Discounted Charges;
Preferred Provider Organizations (PPO)

The amount of money a provider charges for its health services less a fixed discount, which is negotiated between the provider and the managed care plan. *Preferred provider organizations (PPO)* typically seek discounted fee-for-service arrangements with physicians, hospitals, and other providers that are selected for their provider networks.

Disease Staging

See also:
Severity of Illness Index

The practice of classifying patients according to the severity of their illness.

Disenrollment

See also:
Enrollment

Termination, either voluntarily or involuntarily, of an employee's coverage under a group health plan. Voluntary disenrollment occurs when a member quits because he/she simply wants to discontinue coverage under that particular plan. Involuntary disenrollment might occur if a member changes jobs, or if he/she cannot comply with recommended treatment plans, or for gross offenses such as fraud, abuse, or non-payment of premiums or copayments.

Disincentive Plan

See also:
Out-of-Network Services (OON)

A type of health plan in which the level of current benefits is reduced if the member uses a provider that is not in the plan's network of providers. Employers frequently offer a disincentive plan to employees as an alternative to a traditional fee-for-service plan in order to save on health care costs without reducing the current level of benefits.

Dispense as Written (DAW)

See also:
Generic Substitution Program

An instruction from a physician or other practitioner to a pharmacist to dispense a brand-name drug rather than a generic substitution. Because branded drugs are generally more costly than generic drugs, many managed care plans have a *generic substitution program*, which requires the pharmacist to dispense generic substitutions if available in order to hold down costs. In some states, generic substitution progams are mandated. However, most plans also have a DAW provision which allows the physician and/or plan member to request a brand-name drug, thus overriding the plan's generic substitution program. In some cases, the additional expense of the branded drug is absorbed by the plan. In other cases, the member may be required to pay the difference between the generic and the brand-name drugs if either the physician or the member requests this option.

Dispensing Fee

A charge levied by pharmacists and added to the price of a drug, which covers the dispensing pharmacist's pharmaceutical expertise and costs involved in filling the prescription.

Doctor of Osteopathy (D.O.)

See also:
Allopathic;
Osteopathic

A physician trained in osteopathic medicine who may use all of the diagnostic and therapeutic measures of ordinary medicine. In addition, the osteopathic physician (D.O.) is trained in the use of therapeutic manipulation of the musculoskeletal system. D.O.s may be licensed to perform medicine and surgery in all states, are eligible for graduate medical education in either *osteopathic* or *allopathic* programs, and are eligible for reimbursment by Medicare and Medicaid for their services.

Domiciliary Care

See: **Custodial Care**

D

DRG "Creep"

See also:
Upcoding

The unethical practice of coding a patient's DRG category for a more severe diagnosis than actually is indicated by the patient's condition. This usually results in greater reimbursement to the provider. Also known as *upcoding.*

DRG Payment Method

See also:
Diagnosis-Related Group (DRG); DRG Rate

An approach to reimbursing for hospital inpatient services which bases the amount of payment on the *DRG* patient classification system. The DRG payment method is used primarily by Medicare, and also by some insurance carriers and managed care plans.

DRG Rate

See also:
Diagnosis-Related Group (DRG); DRG Payment Method

A fixed dollar amount for reimbursement purposes based on an averaging of costs for all patients in a particular *diagnosis-related group (DRG)* in a baseline year. The DRG rate is adjusted for inflation, economic factors, and bad debts.

Drug Counseling

The practice whereby a pharmacist provides a patient with relevant medical and phamacological information concerning the prescribed drug(s) being dispensed. Many managed care drug benefit programs offer drug counseling services in order to help plan members use their medications more effectively. In some states (e.g., Texas), drug counseling is required by law.

Drug Formulary

See also:
Pharmacy and Therapeutics Committee (P&T)

A restricted list of prescription medications covered under a managed care plan, which are approved for use for specific treatments and dispensed through participating pharmacies to plan members. Many managed care plans use drug formularies as a cost-saving technique. Physicians who participate in managed care plans that use formularies must choose only medicines in the formularies. However, many plans have a provision for the physician to override the formulary and select a non-formulary medication when it is deemed medically necessary for the patient. Drug formularies are developed by a *Pharmacy and Therapeutics Committee (P&T)* composed of both pharmacists and physicians who represent a variety of medical specialties. Formularies are subject to periodic review and modification by the managed care plan.

Drug Price Review (DPR)

See also:
Average Wholesale Prices (AWP);
Blue Book

A monthly updating of drug prices, based on *average wholesale prices (AWP)* derived from the American Druggist's *Blue Book*. Price maximums for drugs are established through the DPR process.

Drug Utilization Management (DUM)

See also:
Counterdetailing;
Drug Utilization Review (DUR);
Provider Profiling;
Utilization Management (UM)

A set of *utilization management* techniques for determining whether a prescribed drug therapy is the most appropriate form of therapy and also which drug is both medically appropriate and financially most cost-effective for the presenting condition. For example, in an attempt to change a physician's prescribing patterns, DUM may use *provider profiling* to detect inappropriate prescribing patterns, and *counterdetailing,* whereby clinical pharmacists inform prescribers about the cost-efficiency and therapeutic efficacy of bioequivalent generic drugs.

Drug Utilization Review (DUR)

See also:
Drug Utilization Management (DUM); Utilization Review (UR)

An evaluation of patterns of physician prescribing, pharmacist dispensing, and targeted customer drug use in order to determine the appropriateness of prescribed drug therapy. DUR is similar to *utilization review (UR)* of medical services and procedures used by managed care plans. DUR involves a range of activities, including prospective, concurrent, and retrospective evaluation of drug use.

Dual Choice (DC)

See also:
Dual Option; Federally Qualified HMO

Usually refers to the federal HMO regulation (Section 1310), which requires any company with 25 or more employees who offers health insurance coverage, pays minimum wage, and whose employees reside in an HMO service area, to offer a *federally qualified HMO* as one of the company's health plan options. However, HMOs must submit a request to the federal government that this option be exercised. Sometimes the term *dual option* is used to describe the federal HMO regulation. Strictly speaking, however, *dual choice* is the more appropriate term when referring to this regulation.

Dual Option

See also:
Dual Choice

Refers to a situation in which an employer contracts with only two health plans, such as an HMO and a traditional indemnity insurance plan, allowing employees to choose one or the other. *Dual option* is similar in meaning to *dual choice* in most respects. The term, *dual choice*, however, is more inclusive in that it also refers to the federal HMO requirement that certain employers must offer an HMO as one of two or more health plan options for employees.

Dues

See also:
Fixed Payment; Premium

Periodic *fixed payments* made by or on behalf of enrollees of a managed care plan, typically an HMO. Dues are comparable to *premiums* in the insurance industry.

Duplicate Coverage Inquiry (DCI)

See also:
Coordination of Benefits (COB);
Duplication of Benefits

A request made by one insurer or group health plan to another in order to determine whether a plan member has duplicate coverage under another plan, that is, *duplication of benefits*. A DCI is made for the purpose of *coordination of benefits (COB),* if necessary.

Duplication of Benefits

See also:
Coordination of Benefits (COB);
Duplicate Coverage Inquiry (DCI);
Primary Payer

Identical or overlapping coverage of an insured person under two or more health care plans. This often occurs when coverage is provided through another plan, such as the spouse's plan. When this situation exists, *coordination of benefits (COB)* usually occurs between the two (or more) plans.

Durable Medical Equipment (DME)

Equipment for use at home required by an individual because of a medical condition. DME devices are designed for repeated (i.e., non-consumable) use, are used primarily and customarily for medical purposes, and generally are not useful to a person in the absence of illness or injury. Examples of DME are: crutches, wheelchairs, hospital beds, and oxygen equipment.

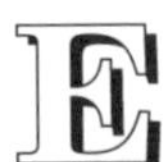

Early and Periodic Screening, Diagnosis, and Treatment (EPSDT)

See also:
Medicaid

A Medicaid program for participants under the age of 21, which pays for screening and diagnostic services to detect physical or mental problems or to provide health care, treatment and other services needed to correct or ameliorate any disabilities or chronic conditions discovered.

Effective Date

See also:
Termination Date

The date a health plan contract becomes in force, as opposed to the *termination date*, which is the date on which a group health contract expires.

Elective Surgery

See also:
Cosmetic Treatment

A surgical procedure for a condition that is not considered an emergency nor life threatening. Such surgery is subject to the choice or decision of the patient and physician. An example is *cosmetic surgery*. Most managed care plans do not cover this type of elective surgery. Hip replacement surgery, on the other hand, is an example of elective surgery that is likely to be covered by a managed care plan.

Electronic Data Interchange (EDI)

See also:
Community Health Management Information System (CHMIS); Management Information System (MIS)

A generic name for electronic, computer-based networks that transmit health care data between participating organizations. Claims can be processed electronically using EDI, eliminating the need to submit claims on paper forms, thereby improving efficiency and saving costs by reducing turnaround time, paperwork and errors. With EDI, providers can receive immediate eligibility verification and authorization on patients from the patients' health plans. An example of EDI is a *Community Health Management Information System (CHMIS)*, which transmits health care data among hospitals, physicians, employers, third party payors within a community.

Element

See also:
Utilization Review (UR)

In a *utilization review (UR),* refers to a component of an audit criterion consisting of a primary indicator or minimum essential evidence that a particular aspect of care has been provided to the plan member.

Eligibility

See also:
Eligible Person

The specific requirements which the members of a group health plan and their dependents must satisfy in order to become insured. Eligibility also refers to a patient's status with respect to medical services that he/she may receive as covered benefits.

Eligibility Date

See also:
Eligibility Period; Waiting Period

The date on which a member of a particular group (e.g., a company's employees) becomes eligible to apply for benefits under the group health plan. For example, a new employee may have to wait for a specified period of time, called the *waiting period* or *eligibility period* (usually thirty days), before becoming eligible to apply for health care coverage under the employer's group plan. The end of that waiting period is defined as the "eligibility date."

Eligibility Period

See also:
Eligibility Date; Evidence of Insurability (E of I)

A specified period of time following the *eligibility date* (usually thirty days) during which a member of particular group (e.g., a company's employees) is eligible to apply for health insurance coverage under a group plan without providing *evidence of insurability (E of I)*. Also called a *waiting period*.

Eligible Employees

See also:
Covered Person; Eligibility

Refers to those members of an employer group who meet the *eligibility* requirements specified in the employer's group health plan contract to qualify for coverage.

Eligible Expense Offset Plan

See: **Maintenance of Benefits Plan (MOB)**

Eligible Expenses

See also:
Covered Services; Usual, Reasonable, and Customary (URC)

Refers to the *usual, reasonable, and customary (URC)* charges, or another agreed upon fee, for health services and supplies covered under a group health plan.

Emergency Care

See also:
Emergi-Center; Emergency Medical Services (EMS); Free-Standing Emergency Medical Services Center

Medical care given for a serious medical condition resulting from injury, sickness or mental illness that arises suddenly and requires immediate care and treatment to avoid jeopardy to the life or health of an individual. Emergency care may be provided in a *free-standing emergency medical services center, emergi-center,* or hospital emergency room. Also called *emergency medical services (EMS).*

Emergency Medical Services (EMS)

See: **Emergency Care**

Emergi-Center

See also:
Emergency Medical Services (EMS); Free-Standing Emergency Medical Service Center

An outpatient health care facility which provides immediate, short-term medical care for minor but urgent medical conditions. Usually, emergi-centers are free-standing, that is, physically, organizationally and financially separate from a hospital. Emergi-centers also may be part of a medical center complex. Sometimes called *urgi-center*.

E

Employee Assistance Professionals Association, Inc. (EAPA)

See also:
Employee Assistance Program (EAP)

A trade association representing the professional interests of practitioners in the *employee assistance program (EAP)* field. EAPA provides its members (7,000 in 1993) networking and educational opportunities, develops training programs for EAP staff, publishes literature to promote a better understanding of EAPs, and serves as an information resource on EAPs.
Address: EAPA, Inc., 4601 N. Fairfax Dr., Suite 1001, Arlington, VA 22203
Phone: (703) 522-6272; Fax: (703) 522-4585

Employee Assistance Program (EAP)

An internal assistance program set up by some employers to help troubled employees (e.g., employees with alcohol or drug abuse problems, family problems, and other behavioral problems) obtain needed treatment. The EAP may be administered internally by trained counselors or by an outside consultant organization. Confidentiality is strictly maintained. Programs may offer counseling, training in coping skills, comprehensive stress management courses, and referrals to outside resources for professional help.

Employee Assistance Society of North America (EASNA)

See also:
Employee Assistance Program (EAP)

A professional organization for *Employee Assistance Program (EAP)* practitioners. EASNA offers its members educational and professional development programs, networking opportunities, and legislative advocacy. The organization has developed a set of EAP standards and offers an EAP accreditation program to purchasers and clients of EAPs in order to promote excellence in EAP programming.
Address: EASNA, 2728 Phillips, Berkley, MI 48072
Phone: (313) 545-3888; Fax: (n/a by request)

E

Employee Benefits Information System (EBIS)

See also:
Bundled Billing; Management Information System (MIS); Unbundling

Specialized software used by third party administrators to administer benefits for employer groups and by employers (typically self-insured) to administer employee benefits in-house. EBIS is used to evaluate utilization data and claims payments to ensure that claims are not overpaid, especially when the cause may be overbilling by providers. For example, EBIS can "unbundle" claims into individual components or "bundle" a group of components into a single procedure. Other functions include: checking billing codes, checking billed procedures against claims history data, and identifying charges that are not "usual and customary," and procedures that are out of line with normal practice.

Employee Benefits Representative (EBR)

An individual employed by an insurance company or managed care organization who is responsible for the sale and service of employee benefit insurance plans, including traditional imdemnity insurance, managed fee-for-service, point-of- service (POS), HMO, and PPO plans.

Employee Benefits Research Institute (EBRI)

A non-profit, non-partisan public policy research organization which provides educational and research materials about employee benefits to employers, employees, retired workers, public officials, members of the press, academics, and the general public. Through books, policy forums, and a monthly subscription service, EBRI contributes to the formulation of effective and responsible employer-sponsored health, welfare, and retirement policies.
Address: EBRI, 2121 K Street, NW, Suite 600
Washington, DC 20037-1896
Phone: (202) 659-0670; Fax: (202) 775-6312

Employee Contribution

See also:
Contributory Plan;
Employer Contribution

In a *contributory plan*, the amount of money that an employee must contribute towards the premium cost of the employer's group health plan. Payments usually are monthly. (Compare with *employer contribution*.)

Employee Retirement Income Security Act (ERISA)

See also:
American Health Security Act of 1993 (AHSA);
Corporate Alliances;
Explanation of Benefits (EOB);
Mandated Benefits

A federal law enacted in 1974 which shields self-insured employers from complying with state-mandated benefits or paying premium taxes (as insurance companies and managed care plans are required to do). ERISA also prevents states from mandating all employers in the state to purchase coverage from health care plans that offer a uniform package of benefits. Another ERISA provision requires that health plans provide an *explanation of benefits* statement describing the benefits under the plan, the persons responsible for operating the plan, the arrangements for funding and amending the plan, and provides information on members' rights of appeal if a claim has been denied. Several of the national health care reform plans would amend ERISA in various ways. For example, the *American Health Security Act of 1993 (AHSA)* modifies ERISA to apply only to corporate alliancesand specifies the benefits package and establishes fiduciary, solvency, and reporting requirements for alliance sponsors. AHSA also modifies the ERISA preemption provision to apply only to employers and health plans in *corporate alliances*.

E

Employer Contribution

See also:
Contributory Plan;
Non-Contributory Plan

The amount of money contributed by the employer toward the premium costs of its group health plan. The amount varies widely among employers and is a critical variable in any risk analysis. Employer contributions can be based on dollar amounts, percentages of premium, employment status, or other variables or combinations of variables. When an employer pays the entire cost of the plan and there is 100% employee participation, the plan is called a *non-contributory plan*.

Employer Eligibility Requirements

See also:
Eligibility

These are conditions of employment set by the employer which must be met by all employees in order to be eligible for group health coverage.

Employer Mandate

See also:
American Health Security Act of 1993 (AHSA); Mandated Benefits; Standard Benefits Package

A federal requirement included in several health care reform proposals whereby every employer would have to pay on behalf of its employees a percentage of the average premium of a *standard benefits package*. For example, under the *American Health Security Act of 1993 (AHSA),* employers would pay 80% of health care premiums for an average cost health plan. Amounts for small employers would have a ceiling, depending on the size of the company and its average wage. Consumers would pay a 20% share of the premium. Self-employed and low-income families would pay a fixed portion of their income. Copayments would be required for office visits and treatments. The federal government would subsidize premiums of low-income families and of some employees of small and medium- size companies. *Employer mandate* also refers to a requirement that all employers must offer at least one health plan to employees, though employers may not necessarily be required to pay for the coverage.

Encounter

See also:
Encounters Per Member Per Year; Follow-Up

The face-to-face meeting of a patient with a provider for evaluation or treatment. Usually, this refers to an outpatient visit. In managed care, if a plan member receives more than one treatment within the same or related department during the same visit, it usually is counted as a single encounter. However, if a member receives treatments from two or more unrelated departments during the same visit, these are counted as multiple encounters. For example, an orthopedic evaluation and an optical examination performed during a single visit to a multispecialty group practice, would be counted as two encounters.

Encounters Per Member Per Year

See also:
Encounter

Refers to the number of encounters experienced by each plan member on a yearly basis. This measurement is used by managed care plans for plan administration and risk analysis. It is calculated as follows: total number of encounters per year divided by the total number of plan members per year.

End Stage Renal Disease (ESRD)

See also:
Renal Dialysis Center

A classification of patients with advanced kidney disease or renal impairment. ERSD virtually always is irreversible and permanent, and requires dialysis or kidney transplantation to ameliorate uremic (blood-kidney) systems and maintain life. Dialysis usually is performed at a *renal dialysis center.*

Enrolled Group

See also:
Eligible Person;
Enrollment

The total number of *eligible persons* with the same employer or membership in the same organization who are enrolled in a group health plan. Usually, group plans have stipulations regarding the minimum size of a group and the minimum percentage of a group that must enroll before the coverage is available.

E

Enrollee

See also:
Member;
Subscriber

Refers to an individual who subscribes to (i.e., is enrolled in) a managed care plan. To be considered an enrollee, the individual must be eligible on his/her own behalf (i.e., not by virtue of being an eligible dependent) to receive the health services under the contract. Also called *member* or *subscriber*.

Enrollment

See also:
Disenrollment;
Enrolled Group;
Open Enrollment

Refers to the total number of covered persons, that is, the *enrolled group*, in a health plan (usually refers to HMOs). Enrollment also may refer to the process by which a health plan signs up individuals and groups for membership, or the number of enrollees who sign up in any one group. The antonym in this case is *disenrollment.*

Entitlement

See also:
Consolidated Omnibus Budget Reconciliation Act of 1985 (COBRA)

Refers to employee benefits that are required by law, such as retention of eligibility for medical benefits by terminated employees under the *Consolidated Omnibus Budget Reconciliation Act of 1985 (COBRA),* also Medicare and Medicaid. Entitlement also refers to the popular perception that long-standing benefits are to some extent a matter of right. For example, many people consider employee health benefits to be an entitlement.

Ergonomic Hazard

See also:
Cumulative Trauma Disorder (CTD); Occupational Hazard; Occupational and Safety Health Act (OSHA); Occupational Safety and Health Administration (OSHA)

An unsafe workplace condition associated with a job process, work method, or work station, generally caused by ineffective design of work station, tools and job. Ergonomic hazards can result in *cumulative trauma disorder (CTD),* injury, or illness to a worker. Examples of ergonomic hazards include: a poorly designed work station which requires awkward postures of the upper body to perform tasks; inappropriate or inadequate hand tools; excessive vibration from power tools; lack of adjustable chairs, footrests, and work surfaces at a work station, etc. The *Occupational Safety and Health Act of 1970 (OSHA)* requires all employers to provide workers with a workplace that is free from recognized serious *occupational hazards*, including ergonomic hazards. The *Occupational Safety and Health Administration (OSHA)* has developed guidelines to help employers meet their responsibilities under OSHA.

Evidence of Coverage See: **Certificate of Coverage (COC)**

Evidence of Insurability (E of I)

See also:
Eligible Person;
Open Enrollment

Refers to proof presented through written statements, such as an application form and/or a medical examination, that an individual is eligible for a certain type of insurance coverage. Evidence of insurability (E of I) is required for *eligible persons* who do not enroll in a group health plan during the *open enrollment* period (usually a 30 day period), or who apply for reinstatement after having previously withdrawn from the plan or after having received an overall maximum benefit, or who apply for excess amounts of group life or disability insurance. Also called "evidence of good health."

Exception

See also:
Element;
Utilization Review (UR)

A clearly defined reason, instance, or circumstance in *utilization review* (UR) which, if documented in the patient's medical record, accounts for the absence (or presence) of an *element* of information in the medical record. An exception also can be alternative secondary evidence that is acceptable to the UR committee.

E

Excess-of-Loss Reinsurance

See also:
Reinsurance;
Stop-Loss Reinsurance

A type of *reinsurance* sold to primary insurers to cover all annual claims above a preset threshold for each covered person. A common threshold is $100,000 per case per year for the typical primary insurance policy's limit of $1 million for each covered person's lifetime. The reinsurer, however, does not cover normal risks that are covered in the primary insurance policy. Thus, its financial exposure is limited to the $1 million cases only. The reinsurer usually sets overall limits of its own. Premiums are set by expected experience (i.e., "experience rated") and are continually renegotiated based on experience. Excess-of-loss reinsurance generally is on a per case basis in contrast to *stop-loss reinsurance*, which usually is written on an aggregate basis and pays all the primary insurer's claims above a cumulative annual amount.

Exclusions

See also:
Cosmetic Surgery;
Pre-Existing Condition

Specific conditions (e.g., *pre-existing conditions*) or circumstances listed in a group health contract or employee benefit plan for which the policy or plan will not provide benefit payments. For example, insurance companies frequently exclude high-risk individuals or families with a history of serious illness or catastrophic injury from coverage under a group plan. Another common exclusion is *cosmetic surgery*.

Exclusive Multiple Option (EMO)

See also:
Exclusive Provider Organization (EPO)

A "single vendor" arrangement whereby an insurance carrier or managed care plan offers an employer a comprehensive package of plans which may include any combination of indemnity insurance, HMO, PPO, or POS plans under the sponsoring plan's management. The employer, in turn, agrees not to enter into an agreement with any other carrier for coverage of eligible employees.

Exclusive Provider Organization (EPO)

See also:
Exclusive Multiple Option (EMO)

A type of managed care plan which provides benefits only if care is rendered by providers with which the plan contracts (with certain exceptions for emergency or out-of-area services). Frequently, exclusive provider organizations (EPO) are offered to large employers because the plans combine features of HMOs (e.g., enrolled population, limited provider panel, gatekeepers, utilization management, capitated provider reimbursement) and PPOs (e.g., flexible benefit design, negotiated fees, fee-for-service payments, experience rating). In an EPO arrangement, employers agree not to enter into an agreement with any other plan or insurance carrier for coverage of eligible employees. In turn, the EPO provides coverage only for services provided by contracted providers. Technically, many HMOs can be considered EPOs; however, EPOs are regulated under insurance statutes rather than federal and state HMO regulations.

Expected Claims

See also:
Experience Rating;
Rating Process

Refers to the projected level of claims of a covered person or group for a defined contract period. The level of expected claims is also known as a desired loss ratio, or "break even point," relative to the projected premium. Insurance companies and managed care plans use this estimation for setting rates using an *experience rating* methodology.

Expedited Appeal

See also:
Appeal

An initial request by telephone for additional review of a utilization review organization's determination not to certify an admission, extension of stay, or other health care service. Sometimes called *reconsideration.*

Experience Rating

See also:
Community Rating;
Expected Claims;
Prospective Rating

A rate-setting methodology whereby health plan premiums are adjusted to reflect the claims experience of a specific subscriber group. The needed revenues are then projected for a future policy year for that group, based on the *expected claims*. There are two types of experience rating: prospective and retrospective. In *prospective rating*, the premium includes expected costs of health services, plus a margin for higher than anticipated claims, as well as expenses and profit. For large employers, the margin, expenses, and profit usually are negotiated annually with the insurer. Retrospective experience rating allows the insurer to refund some or all of the difference between claims expenses and paid premiums after the period of coverage has passed.

Experience Refund

See also:
Expected Claims;
Experience Rating

A provision in most group health plans that use an experience rating methodology for the return of some portion of the premium to the policyholder because of lower-than-*expected claims*.

Experience-Rated Premium

See also:
Community Rating; Expected Claims; Experience Rating

A health insurance premium based on the *expected claims* experience of, or utilization of services by, a contract group according to the group's age, sex, and any other attributes expected to affect the group's health care utilization. An experience-rated premium is subject to periodic adjustment based on actual claims or utilization experience of the covered group. The opposite of an experience-rated premium is one that is set using a *community rating* methodology.

Experimental Procedures

See also:
Alternative Therapies

Health care services (e.g., medical, surgical, psychiatric, substance abuse, or other services, supplies, treatments, procedures, drug therapies, devices, etc.) which a health plan has determined to be unproven by scientific evidence or not generally accepted by informed health care professionals in the U.S. as effective in treating the condition, illness, or diagnosis for which their use is proposed. Generally, experimental procedures are not covered under managed care plans.

Expiration Date

See also:
Eligibility Date; Master Group Contract

This may be either the date on which the health insurance *master group contract* expires or the date that an individual or employee ceases to be eligible for coverage under a group health plan.

Explanation of Benefits (EOB)

See also:
Employee Retirement Income Security Act (ERISA)

A statement sent by a managed care plan or an insurance company to a plan member who files a claim. The explanation of benefits (EOB) lists the services provided, the amount billed, and the payment made. The EOB statement must also explain why a claim was or was not paid, and provide information about the individual's rights of appeal. EOB statements are required under *ERISA*. Sometimes called *explanation of medical benefits (EOMB)*.

Extended Benefits

See also:
Extension of Benefits

The term can refer to comprehensive benefits provided in excess of basic health care plans. It also can mean *extension of benefits* for limited periods after termination of plan coverage.

Extended Care Facility (ECF)

See also:
Nursing Home;
Skilled Nursing Facility (SNF)

A *nursing home* or *skilled nursing facility (SNF)* licensed to provide 24-hour nursing care for patients who do not require the full care provided by a hospital, but their medical or physical condition renders the patients unable to care for themselves. Often, ECFs are associated with hospitals, but provide care at a lower cost. Such a facility may offer skilled, intermediate, or custodial care, or any combination of these levels of care. Most health plans exclude extended coverage in an ECF unless the facility provides specific rehabilitation services that will result in the patient's eventual discharge.

Extension of Benefits

See also:
COBRA;
Continuation of Coverage;
Extended Benefits;
Termination Date

A provision of many insurance policies which allows medical coverage to continue past the policy's termination date for employees not actively at work and for dependents hospitalized on the *termination date.* Such extended coverage usually applies only to the specific medical condition which has caused the disability. Coverage continues only until the employee returns to work or the dependent leaves the hospital. Extension of benefits is not as common since the implementation of *COBRA* regulations because COBRA has a provision for *continuation of coverage.*

External Evaluation

See also:
Pre-established Criteria

Refers to an independent appraisal of a program's performance against measurable *pre-established criteria*. External evaluations usually are conducted by individuals who are not affiliated with either the program's sponsor or the activity under evaluation. Sometimes called *external review*.

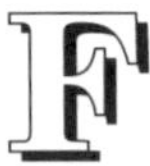

Factored Rating

See: **Adjusted Community Rating (ACR)**

Faculty Practice Plan (FPP)

See also:
Independent Practice Association (IPA)

A type of corporate health plan (managed care or fee-for-service) organized around a teaching program, primarily at university hospitals. A faculty practice plan (FFP) may be a single physician group, which includes all the physicians providing services to patients at a teaching hospital and clinics, or it may include multiple groups drawn along specialty lines, such as psychiatry, cardiology or surgery. Health plans generally contract with the legal group representing the FFP rather than with the individual physicians within the FFP.

Family Deductible

See also:
Calendar Year;
Deductible

A *deductible* that is satisfied by the combined expenses of all covered family members. For example, a program with a $100 deductible may limit its application to a maximum of three deductibles, or $300, for the entire family regardless of the number of family members. In this example, a family of four or more would pay no more than a total of $300 in deductibles each *calendar year*.

Family Practice (FP)

See also:
Gatekeeper;
General Practitioner (GP);
Primary Care Physician (PCP)

A type of primary care practice which is directed at the whole family. The family practice physician is a generalist, or *general practitioner (GP)*, who has completed a three-year accredited residency and cares for patients of all ages with a variety of medical conditions. Family practitioners (both M.D.s and D.O.s) often serve as *gatekeepers* for managed care plans (typically HMOs) with responsibility for managing the clinical care provided to plan members.

Favored Nations Discount

A contractual term of agreement included in some managed care contracts which states that the provider will automatically give the payor the best discount given to anyone else. The favored nations discount clause commonly is found in contracts between Blue Cross plans and participating hospitals.

Federal Employee Health Benefits Program (FEHBP)

See also:
Office of Personnel Management (OPM)

A large government health care program which provides health benefits to federal employees. The FEHBP is administered by the *Office of Personnel Management (OPM)*, a federal agency with which managed care plans contract to provide needed health care services to federal employees.

Federally Qualified HMO (FQHMO)

See also:
Health Maintenance Organization (HMO)

A prepaid managed care plan which has applied for and has met federal qualification requirements for HMOs. Federal qualification regulations include the following standards: 1) stipulation of health services offered; 2) community rating (with some flexibility); 3) a board of directors of which one-third are HMO members; 4) health education; 5) social services; 6) fiscal viability; 7) a quality assurance program; and 8) an enrollment that is broadly representative of the general population of the HMO service area. The HMO Amendments Act of 1988 generated new regulations that allowed FQHMOs greater flexibility in their product offerings. For example, FQHMOs now are allowed to offer other managed care products, such as a PPO, a POS (with some restrictions), and a competitively priced non-federally qualified managed care plan. Some HMOs elect not to be federally qualified even though they meet all of the qualifying requirements. Usually this is due to the amount of paperwork associated with the qualifying process.

Federation of American Health Systems (FAHS)

A trade association representing the investor-owned hospital and health care systems industry, consisting of more than 1,400 institutions in all 50 states, the District of Columbia, Puerto Rico, and 11 foreign nations. The primary function of the FAHS is to advocate members' interests to Congress, the Executive Branch, the media, academia, and the public. The FAHS also serves as a clearinghouse for vital information on health care issues and industry positions, policies, and statistics. FAHS conducts research on various health issues, prepares position papers and other informational literature, and offers educational opportunities through an Annual Conference and Business Exposition and through its publications, including the bimonthly Health Systems Review, biweeekly Hotline newsletter of Washington events, monthly newsletter, State-to-State, reporting on legislative and regulatory events. FAHS supports market-based health care reform through managed competition instead of global budgets or price controls.
Address: FAHS, 1111 19th Street, NW, Suite 402, Washington DC 20036
Phone: (202) 833-3090; Fax: (202) 861-0063

F

Fee Allowance Schedule

See: **Fee Schedule** and **Fee Maximum**

Fee Maximum (Fee Max)

See also:
Fee Schedule

The maximum amount that a provider participating in a PPO will be paid for a specific service provided to a plan member under a specific contract. Fee maximums are specified in the *fee schedule.*

Fee Schedule

See also:
Fee Schedule Payment Program;
Scheduled Plan

A comprehensive listing of accepted fees or established allowances which a health plan uses to reimburse a provider on a fee-for-service basis for specified medical procedures. The fee schedule is usually based on CPT billing codes. Sometimes called a *fee allowance schedule.*

Fee Schedule Payment Program

See also:
Fee Maximum;
Scheduled Plan

A reimbursement program in which the plan pays either submitted charges or a *fee maximum*, whichever is less, for any given covered medical service or procedure.

Fee-for-Service Equivalency

See also:
Capitation;
Fee-for-Service Reimbursement (FFS)

A quantitative measure defined as the difference between the amount a provider receives from a managed care reimbursement method, such as *capitation*, compared to *fee-for-service reimbursement (FFS),* characteristic of traditional indemnity insurance.

F

Fee-for-Service Insurance

See also:
Claims Pooling;
Fee-for-Service Reimbursement (FFS)

The traditional type of health insurance in which the insured is reimbursed for covered expenses without regard to choice of provider. Payment up to a stated limit may be made either to the individual incurring and claiming the expense or directly to providers. Premiums, or prepaid amounts of money, are paid to an insurance company by the insured individual or group. The insurer is willing to underwrite the risk of actuarially unexpected losses because by pooling a large number of cases (*claims pooling*), it can normally make the aggregate risk acceptably predictable, though random variation remains. Also called *indemnity insurance* or *traditional indemnity insurance.*

Fee-for-Service Reimbursement (FFS)

See also:
Cost-Based Reimbursement; Fee-for-Service Insurance

A method of reimbursement to providers for each unit of service or procedure performed, including professional service, laboratory, X-Ray, injections, etc. Unlike managed care, which has some cost containment features, fee-for-service reimbursement (FFS) is considered the *traditional indemnity* or *cost-based reimbursement* payment system under which providers receive a payment that does not exceed their billed charges for each unit of service.

Field Underwriting

See also:
Employee Benefits Representative (EBR)

The process of screening prospective buyers of a health plan's products in order to ensure profitable contracting. Typically, this is done by the plan's sales representative, called an *employee benefits representative (EBR)*. Field underwriting may also include authority to quote premium rates of specific products for defined types and sizes of groups.

Filter

See also:
Utilization Management (UM)

A *utilization management* tool used by insurance companies and managed care organizations to try to limit the use of medical resources. A filter might be, for example, a certain fee in a fee-for-service reimbursement system, or the scheduling systems in HMOs.

Financial Accounting Standards - Rule 106 (FAS-106)

A recently adopted (1992) federal rule of the Financial Accounting Standards Board (FASB) which requires employers to show as a liability any financial benefits promised to retired employees if the company fails to set aside enough money to cover these costs during an employee's active working years. The rule covers retiree health and life insurance costs. FAS-106 requires an accounting change for many large corporations. It also allows companies to either take a one-time deduction in earnings or spread out the impact of the accounting change over a twenty-year period.

First Dollar Coverage

Refers to medical expenses covered by a health plan that has no deductibles. In other words, the plan pays a specified percentage of total medical expenses, starting with the "first dollar," rather than a percentage of remaining expenses after the deductible is paid.

Fiscal Intermediary (FI)

See also:
Health Insuring Organization (HIO); Third Party Payor

An insurance company or other private contractor, such as a third party administrator, that collects premiums and pays claims. Fiscal intermediaries are often referred to as *third party payors* because they are not directly involved in the provision of care.

Fixed Payment

See also:
Dues; Premium

A type of *premium* income (i.e., *dues*) which an HMO receives from its members. Dues are fixed per time period and usually paid on a monthly basis, regardless of the amount of covered services received by enrollees.

F

Flexible Benefit Plan (Flex Plan)

See also:
Cafeteria Plan; Section 125 Plan

A type of benefit program offered by some employers, which gives employees the opportunity to select the type of benefits and level of coverage desired from a menu of health plan options. Thus, employees can tailor benefits to their specific needs. By comparison, a traditional benefit plan offers all employees the same benefits and the same level of coverage. A flex plan that is designed in accordance with Section 125 of the Internal Revenue Code is legally known as a *Section 125 plan* or *cafeteria plan* because it allows an employee to choose between cash and several non-taxable benefits, such as group life or medical insurance.

Focused Review

See also:
Utilization Review (UR)

A type of *utilization review* process which identifies and concentrates utilization management resources on certain providers, services, diagnoses and/or geographic areas when the need for utilization controls has been documented. A focused review may be done either in lieu of or prior to a more comprehensive review.

Follow-Up

See also:
Encounter;
Office Visit

Generally, a brief study or review of the problems uncovered in a patient's medical evaluation to determine whether the corrective actions have alleviated the medical problems.

Force Majeure Clause

A clause usually included in most contracts between payors and providers which relieves a party of responsibility if an event occurs beyond its control. For example, if a provider is no longer able to provide services as specified in the managed care contract, the force majeure clause states that the provider is not obligated to fulfill its contract responsibilities.

Formal Grievance Procedure

See also:
Grievance

A formal administrative process used by managed care plans for resolving complaints whereby a plan member or a participating provider can submit complaints to the plan and seek resolutions. The procedure typically consists of filing a formal *grievance*, followed by an investigation, appeal and review, a formal hearing, arbitration (where allowed by the state), an appeal to government agencies, and, as a last resort, a lawsuit. State and federal regulations require HMOs to have clearly defined member grievance procedures. Formal grievance procedures are usually required in insurance and self-funded plans, too.

Formula Approach

See also:
Norms;
Rating Process;
Standards

The use of quantitative *standards* or *norms* that have been established by a managed care plan for evaluating health care services in order to screen out and disallow excessive costs. A formula approach is frequently used by claims processors in rate reviews.

Formulary

See: **Drug Formulary**

F

Foundation for Medical Care (FMC)

See also:
Physician-Hospital Organization (PHO); Prepaid Group Practice Plan

A non-profit, physician-sponsored organization which acquires the business and clinical assets of a physician group and then handles all business management for both parties, physicians and foundation. The FMC usually offers managed care plans a fee schedule for medical services provided by physician members. Most FMCs offer peer review and may contract with third-party administrators for these services. Some FMCs also provide prospective and concurrent utilization review services, similar to commercial utilization review organizations. Some FMCs develop *Physician-Hospital Organizations (PHO)* with hospitals. FMCs often are sponsored by medical societies. Also called *medical foundation*.

Fraud

An intentional misrepresentation of the truth for the purpose of deceiving another person, which causes damage of some sort.

F

Free Choice

See also:
Fee-for-Service Insurance

A health plan provision that permits the plan member to choose any licensed provider rather than restricting the choice to a provider who participates in a plan's provider network. Free choice is generally found in traditional indemnity, or *fee-for-service insurance* plans.

Free-Standing Emergency Medical Services Center

See also:
Emergi-Center; Urgent Care

An outpatient health care facility which is physically, organizationally, and financially separate from a hospital and provides immediate, short-term medical care for minor but urgent medical conditions. Sometimes called *emergi-center, urgi-center,* or *urgent care center*.

Free-Standing Outpatient Surgery Center

See also:
Day Surgery;
Surgi-Center

A health care facility that is physically separate from a hospital and provides prescheduled surgical services on an outpatient basis, generally at a lower cost than inpatient hospital care. Also called *surgi-center*.

Full Time Equivalent (FTE)

A method of counting an organization's staff by classifying an FTE as the equivalent of one full-time employee. For example, two part-time staff members who each work 20 hours per week together equal one FTE.

Funding Level

See also:
Funding Method;
Self-Funded Plan

The amount of revenue required to finance a group health care plan. The funding level for an insured program usually is the premium rate. Under a *self-funded plan,* the funding level often is assessed according to the expected claims costs, plus the stop-loss premium, and all related fees.

Funding Method

See also:
Risk Sharing;
Self-Funded Plan

Refers to the way an employer pays for its employee benefits plan. Several funding methods are used. Some shift risk from the employer to a carrier. Others enable an employer to self-fund its health plan. The most common funding methods are: prospective and/or retrospective premium payments, refunding products, self-funding, and *risk sharing* arrangements.

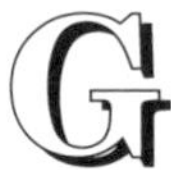

G

Gatekeeper

See also:
Primary Care Physician / Practitioner (PCP)

A *primary care physician (PCP)* or non-physician practitioner who is responsible for managing a plan member's medical treatment, including all referrals for specialty care, ancillary services, and hospital services, throughout the duration of the contract. The gatekeeper is a popular cost-control component of many managed care plans. Managed care plans may offer their gatekeepers financial incentives to limit referrals to specialists for more costly, specialized treatments.

General Hospital

See also:
Specialty Hospital

A medical facility that provides diagnostic and therapeutic inpatient services, both surgical and non-surgical, to patients who have any of a variety of medical conditions. (Contrast with *specialty hospital.*)

General Practitioner (GP)

See also:
Family Practice (FP); Primary Care Physician

A *primary care physician* who cares for individuals and families, regardless of the age or sex of family members. A general practitioner has graduated from an accredited medical school and has completed an accredited residency program.

Generic Drug

See also:
Chemical Equivalents; Generic Substitution Program

A prescription drug which is a *chemical equivalent* copy of a brand-name drug that has an expired patent. Generic drugs are usually less expensive than branded drugs and are sold by their chemical formula, or "generic" name. For example, the brand name for a popular tranquilizer is Valium, but a *chemical equivalent* is also available under the generic name "diazepam." Also called *generic equivalents.*

Generic Substitution Program

See also:
Chemical Equivalents; Generic Drug

A cost-containment program frequently used by managed care plans (also mandated in some states, e.g. Massachusetts) in which the pharmacist contacts physicians who may have prescribed a brand-name drug for a plan member and obtains authorization to substitute a *generic drug* which is a *chemical equivalent* of the branded drug. Proposals for generic substitutions are usually reviewed prior to making the substitution to ensure that risks and benefits are considered.

Geographic Multiplier

See also:
Geographic Practice Cost Index (GPCI)

A mathematical multiplier used for making geographic adjustments to the Medicare fee schedule. Geographic multipliers usually are based on a *geographic practice cost index (GPCI).*

Geographic Practice Cost Index (GPCI)

See also:
Geographic Multiplier; Medicare Economic Index (MEI)

An index which summarizies the prices of inputs to physician services in a geographical area relative to national average prices. The GPCI is used by HCFA for physician price comparisons related to Medicare reimbursement.

Global Budget

A feature of several national health care reform proposals under consideration by U.S. legislators whereby the federal government would impose a national budget on the total amount spent on health care services in the United States. The purpose of a global budget would be to restrain the growth in health care costs by setting annual targets for health care expenditures. However, to be effective, it is thought that global budgets will need to be accompanied by price controls and some constraints on utilization, rather than allowing market forces to determine the allocation of health care resources.

Global Fee

See also:
Bundled Billing;
Coronary Bypass Artery Graft Project (CABG);
Follow-Up;
Unbundling

A method of setting payment rates on an all-inclusive basis. Global fees often are developed by managed care plans (also by Medicaid in some states, such as Massachusetts) for specialty procedures to protect against *unbundling* of claims. For example, for surgery, the surgeon typically conducts a preoperative consultation, then performs the actual surgery, and provides post-surgery *follow-up*. Each of these services can have a separate charge. Likewise, obstetrical services generally include prenatal, delivery, and postnatal care. Because the same physician (or several physicians in a medical group practice) is performing all the services associated with either the surgery or the obstetrical care, the managed care plan negotiates an all-inclusive global fee to discourage the physician(s) from billing for these services separately.

Grace Period

See also:
Lapse;
Renewal

A set number of days past the due date of a premium payment during which medical coverage may not be cancelled and through which the premium payment may be made without penalties. The grace period varies by contract, and is generally 30, 60, 90, or 120 days.

Grievance

See also:
Formal Grievance Procedure

A formal complaint (verbal or written) concerning a person, service, quality of care, or contractual coverage issue, which formally demands resolution by the health plan. Grievances may be submitted by plan members or participating providers to plan administrators as a means to air complaints, seek remedies, or request review of supplemental benefits.

Gross Domestic Product (GDP)

See also:
Gross National Product (GNP);
National Health Expenditures (NHE)

A statistical indicator used by the federal government since 1991 for tracking economic activity in the United States. The GDP measures the total goods and services produced within the U.S., excluding all imports, regardless of ownership, whether foreign or domestic. The government believes that the GDP is a better barometer to use in comparing U.S. economic activity with that of our trading partners than the *gross national product (GNP),* which was used previously. Currently, the GNP is larger than the GDP because U.S. companies earn more abroad than foreign-owned companies earn here. *National health expenditures (NHE)* usually are expressed as a percentage of GDP (since 1991). For example, in 1993, health care spending accounted for more than 14% of the GDP (estimated at $940 billion), up from 13.3% in 1991.

Gross National Product (GNP)

See also:
Gross Domnestic Product (GDP);
National Health Expenditures (NHE)

A statistical indicator used by the federal government to track national economic activity. GNP measures the total output of goods and services by U.S. companies, including profits on U.S. operations abroad. Unlike the *gross domestic product (GDP)*, the GNP does not include profits of foreign-owned companies operating within the U.S. Prior to 1991, government estimates of *national health expenditures (NHE)* were expressed as a percentage of GNP. Since 1991, NHE has been presented as a percentage of GDP, which is believed to be a better barometer to use in comparing U.S. economic activity with that of our trading partners. GNP reports still are being produced by the federal government, but will gradually assume a lesser role.

Group Contract

See also:
Master Group Contract

An insurance contract for group benefits made with an employer or other entity under which a number of employees and their dependents, or members of a homogeneous group, such as a union, are insured under a single policy.

Group Health Association of America, Inc. (GHAA)

A trade association representing the interests of HMOs in policy and legislative issues affecting the managed care industry. GHAA had 350 HMO members in 1993. In addition to HMO organizational membership, GHAA offers individual, student, international, corporate supporting memberships, and memberships for state managed care associations. GHAA provides legislative representation at federal and state levels, legal counsel, educational programs, research, and publications. The organization also maintains a library of managed care resources, which is open to members and non-members. GHAA publications include the annual National Directory of HMOs and HMO Industry Profile, a bimonthly HMO Magazine, and a biweekly *HMO Managers Letter*.
Address: GHAA, 1129 20th St., NW, Suite 600, Washington, DC 20036
Phone: (202) 778-3200; Fax: (202) 331-7487

G

Group Insurance

See: **Group Contract**

Group Model HMO

See also:
Health Maintenance Organization (HMO); Multispecialty Group (MSG)

A type of HMO which contracts with large, *multispecialty groups* of physicians for health care services for its enrollees. Typically, the group model HMO provides the facility, non-physician clinical staff, and administrative support for the medical group. The HMO also is responsible for contracting with hospitals for care of its patients. Usually a group model HMO compensates its physicians at a negotiated fixed or capitated rate. Participating physicians also may enter into various profit-sharing arrangements with the HMO.

Group Practice

See also:
Group Practice Without Walls (GPWW); Multispecialty Group (MSG)

A group of physicians organized as a professional, not-for-profit corporation and engaged in the coordinated practice of their profession. Members may share facilities, common overhead expenses, medical records, substantial portions of the equipment, as well as professional, technical, and administrative staff. In some cases, group practice physicians also share earnings. Physicians involved in a group practice may represent a single specialty or a range of specialties (i.e., *multispecialty group practice).*

Group Practice Without Walls (GPWW)

See: **Clinic Without Walls (CWW)**

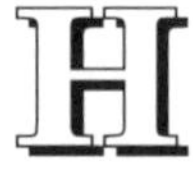

HCFA 1500

A standard, universal billing form developed by HCFA for physicians and other practitioners to use for billing professional fees to health insurance carriers.

HCFA Common Procedural Coding System (HCPCS)

See also:
Current Procedural Terminology (CPT)

An alphanumeric coding system for reporting physician and other provider services, procedures, and supplies to Medicare patients. HCPCS includes *Current Procedural Terminology (CPT)* codes, and also national and local codes. Five-digit codes beginning with A through V are national; codes beginning with W through Z are local. The national codes supplement CPT codes and include physician services not in the CPT, as well as non-physician services, like ambulance, physical therapy, and durable medical equipment (DME). Local codes are developed by local Medicare carriers to supplement the national codes.

HCFA Rate Cell Verification

See also:
Capitation;
Rate Cells

HCFA assigns all Medicare beneficiaries to certain *capitation* rate groups, called *rate cells*. HCFA's rate cell verification process involves confirming the criteria which HCFA uses (e.g., age, sex, geographical location, economic status) to assign Medicare beneficiaries to a particular rate cell.

Health Alliance

See also:
American Health Security Act of 1993 (AHSA);
Corporate Alliance;
Health Insurance Purchasing Cooperative (HIPC);
Managed Competition;
Regional Health Alliance

A large pool of businesses and consumers formed for the purpose of negotiating prices for health benefits with networks of physicians, hospitals, insurers and other health care providers. Health alliances are a key feature of President Clinton's proposed health care reform plan, *American Health Security Act of 1993 (AHSA),* and are similar to *health insurance purchasing cooperatives (HIPC)* in the *managed competition* model. The AHSA plan would create a nationwide system of *regional* and *corporate health alliances* to strengthen consumer bargaining power and spread risks. Each state would decide how many alliances to set up. Companies with fewer than 5,000 employees would be required to join a health alliance in their area. Joining would be optional, however, for the very large employers. Health alliances would have broad regulatory powers to collect money from employers, negotiate contracts with health plans, and enforce caps on health insurance premiums.

Health and Human Services Department (HHS)

See also:
Health Care Financing Administration (HCFA); Office of Prepaid Health Care Operations & Oversight (OPHCOO)

A federal Cabinet level agency which oversees government health care programs and activities, including Social Security, Medicare, and Medicaid. The *Health Care Financing Administration (HCFA), Health Resources & Services Administration (HRSA),* and *Office of Prepaid Health Care Operations & Oversight (OPHCOO)* (formerly known as the *Office of Health Maintenance Organizations)* are part of the HHS, which once was named the Health, Education and Welfare Department (HEW).
Address: HHS, 200 Independence Ave., SW, Washington, DC 20201
Phone: (202) 619-0257; Fax: *(by department)*

Health Care Coalition

See also:
Business Coalition

A consortium of local employers, providers, and sometimes third party payors generally formed for the purpose of controlling health care costs and enhancing the efficiency of health care delivery while also maintaining quality. Health care coalitions are cooperative partnerships that tend to represent wider interests and have broader agendas than employer- only *business coalitions*. For example, the Greater Cleveland Coalition is attempting to assess quality of care by measuring clinical outcomes and patient satisfaction. The top-rated providers are rewarded with increased business from coalition members. Some coalitions focus primarily on public policy issues affecting health care. Others set community education and outreach as a priority, while still others focus on community access to health care, including care for the unemployed, the uninsured, and the indigent.

Health Care Financing Administration (HCFA)

See also:
Health and Human Services Department (HHS);
Medicaid;
Medicare

The federal agency responsible for administering *Medicare* and overseeing states' administration of *Medicaid*. HCFA also manages HMO qualification, the Utilization and Quality Control Peer Review, and a variety of other health care financing and quality assurance programs. HCFA is a part of the *Health and Human Services Department (HHS)*. HCFA's main office is in Washington, DC. The agency also has a Research Office and an Office of Statistics & Data Management, both located in Baltimore, Maryland.
Main office phone: (202) 727-0735
Research Office phone: (410) 966-6674
Office of Statistics & Data Mgmt. phone: (410) 597-3855

Health Care Plan (HCP)

See also:
Managed Care Plan (MCP)

An agreement whereby a prepaid health care contractor either furnishes health care services (e.g., hospitalization, surgery, medical or nursing care, drugs, other restorative appliances) or reimburses other providers for such care to plan members. Members of the health care plan pay the contractor stipulated premiums, usually on a monthly basis. The contractor may be a medical organization, a non-profit organization, an insurer, or a self-funded employer that can meet the state's requirements.

Health Care Prepayment Plan (HCPP)

See also:
Medicare;
Medicare Risk Contract

A type of cost-reimbursed, prepaid health plan for *Medicare* beneficiaries (as opposed to a *Medicare risk contract*). HCPPs are reimbursed by HCFA for the reasonable cost of services actually provided to Medicare enrollees. Unlike HMOs and competitive medical plans (CMP), HCPPs are relatively unregulated. For example, HCPPs are not required to have open enrollment. Also, HCPPs do not have to provide the full range of Medicare-covered services, nor are they responsible for emergency care, nor must they provide any rights of appeal to members. Any managed care organization that provides services to enrolled members through its own staff or through contracted providers may become a HCPP. Many HCPPs are labor or employer organizations that arrange for provision of services exclusively to their members.

Health Care Quality Improvement Act of 1986 (HCQIA)

See also:
National Practitioner Data Bank (NPDB);
Peer Review Organization (PRO)

A federal regulation which ensures antitrust immunity for peer review activities. To participate in the HCQI, a hospital or health plan must report to a national clearinghouse, called the *National Practitioner Data Bank (NPDB),* any actions taken to restrict or terminate the privileges of a physician. Hospitals and health plans must check with the NPDB regarding a physician's record at the time of appointment to their medical staff or change of privileges. If the provider or the plan fails to check the NPDB, it may incur a liability risk if the physician's practice comes into question at a later date.

Health History

See also:
Evidence of Insurability (E of I)

A form used by health plan underwriters for evaluating the medical history of individuals who apply for coverage in order to determine acceptable risk. Physicians and other practitioners also obtain a health history on a patient at the time of a physicial examination.

Health Insurance Association of America (HIAA)

A national trade association for commercial health insurers. HIAA serves as a forum for public policy development, represents members' views to Congress, state legislatures, and the public, and influences legislation and regulations. HIAA also conducts research, publishes literature and policy analyses on health insurance trends, and advises members about pertinent government activities and public opinion on health care issues. A managed care advocacy network was developed in 1991 to cultivate the managed care environment. A Managed Care Resource Center serves as a clearinghouse for publications and materials on managed care. Other membership services include: networking opportunities, educational seminars, workshops, publications (e.g., Source Book of Health Insurance Data), on-line database information services, and a consumer helpline.
Address: HIAA, 1025 Connecticut Ave., NW, Washington, DC 20036-3998
Phone: (202) 223-7800; Fax: (202) 223-7897

Health Insurance Network (HIN)

See also:
Health Insurance Purchasing Cooperative (HIPC);
Managed Competition;
Regional Health Alliance

A proposed health care reform mechanism for pooling the health care purchasing power of small employers. The Health Insurance Network (HIN) concept was part of President Bush's "Comprehensive Health Reform Program." HINs would enable small firms to purchase lower cost health insurance by reducing the administrative costs and by exempting insurance purchased from the HINs from excessive state mandates, anti-managed care laws, and premium taxes. HINs are similar to *health insurance purchasing cooperatives (HIPCs)* proposed by the Jackson Hole Group in their *managed competition* model and the *regional health alliances* in President Clinton's health care reform plan.

Health Insurance Program (HI)

See also:
Medicare

The compulsory part (Part A) of the *Medicare* program which covers inpatient hospitalization costs (currently reimbursed using the DRG system) and post-hospital care. The HI program (also called *Medicare Part A)* also pays for pharmaceuticals provided in hospitals, but not for drugs provided in outpatient settings.

Health Insurance Purchasing Cooperative (HIPC)

See also:
Health Alliance; Health Insurance Network (HIN); Managed Competition

A proposed collective health insurance purchasing agent which would act on behalf of small employers and individuals for purchasing group health benefits. The HIPC is a key component of the Jackson Hole Group's *managed competition* model for a reformed health care system. HIPCs would spread and manage risk, take advantage of economies of scale, and reduce administrative costs. The HIPC concept is similar to the *health insurance network (HIN)* idea for small employers, which was considered by President Bush, and the *health alliance* concept in President Clinton's health care reform plan. The main difference between these proposed agencies is that HIPCs and health alliances would act on behalf of both individuals and small employers, whereas HIN would have acted on behalf of small employers only.

Health Insurance Standards Board (HISB)

See also:
Health Insurance Purchasing Cooperative (HIPC); Managed Competition; National Health Board (NHB); Outcomes Management Standards Board (OMSB)

One of three proposed private sector organizations which would be created under the *managed competition* model for health care reform, developed by the Jackson Hole Group. The HISB would advise on health insurance coverage issues, insurance market competition, accountability, underwriting, business practices that serve the small business market, and integration of state laws and regulations under a managed competition system. Members of the HISB would be selected from insurance, employer, and consumer groups.

Health Insuring Organization (HIO)

See also:
Fiscal Intermediary (FI); Medicaid

A type of prepaid managed care plan for Medicaid beneficiaries in which states contract with organizations exclusively dedicated to serving a Medicaid population. HIOs initially were statewide or regional *fiscal intermediaries (FI)* that contracted with the state Medicaid agency to receive capitation payments. HIOs then paid providers on a fee-for- service basis. In some states, HIOs are mandatory programs as opposed to voluntary enrollment programs offered by Medicaid HMOs. However, in 1985, Congress ruled that HIOs must meet the same enrollment rules as HMOs for mix of commercial and Medicaid enrollment. Because an HIO contracts with state Medicaid agencies and is not a commercial HMO, it cannot meet this requirement. Thus, further development of mandatory HIOs has ceased.

Health Maintenance Organization (HMO)

See also:
Group Model HMO;
IPA Model HMO;
Network Model HMO;
Staff Model HMO

A comprehensive health care financing and delivery organization which provides or arranges for provision of health care services to enrollees within a geographicaal area through a panel of providers. Enrollees pay a fixed, prepaid amount of money regardless of the amount of actual services used. HMOs offer coverage for preventive services and use primary care physicians as *gatekeepers*. Four types of HMO models are common: 1) *staff model* in which physicians are salaried employees of the HMO; 2) *IPA model,* which contracts with Independent Practice Associations (IPA), which, in turn, contract with independent physicians who practice in their own offices; 3) *group model,* which contracts with multispecialty physician group practices; 4) *network model,* which contracts with two or more independent group practices and/or IPAs.

Health Outcomes Institute (HOI)

See also:
InterStudy;
Outcomes Management System (OMS);
Outcomes Measurement;
Outcomes Research

A privately funded health policy think tank, organized in February, 1993, which specializes in *outcomes research*. HOI is continuing to develop and distribute the *Outcomes Management System (OMS)* methodology for measuring outcomes, which originally was developed by *InterStudy*, a health care research organization. The OMS measures patient function, well-being, and clinical status. OMS methodology relies on quality-of-life self-assessments by patients who complete a questionnaire and condition-specific clinical forms completed by physicians.
Address: HOI, 2001 Killebrew Dr., Suite 122, Bloomington, MN 55425
Phone: (612) 858-9188; Fax: (612) 858-9189

H

Health Plan Employer Data and Information Set (HEDIS)

See also:
National Committee for Quality Assurance (NCQA);
HMO Group, The

A standard data reporting system developed in 1991 by *The HMO Group*, several major employers, and Towers Perrin, an employer benefits consulting firm, to measure the quality and performance of health plans nationwide. A key goal HEDIS, which is being tested in a pilot project by 17 HMOs, is to standardize health plan performance measures. HEDIS focuses on four aspects of health care: 1) quality; 2) access and patient satisfaction; 3) membership and utilization; and 4) finance. Within each focus area is a set of specific measures. For example, quality assessments focus on preventive medicine, prenatal care, acute and chronic disease, and mental health. Finance measures focus on rates, indicators of financial stability, liquidity indicators, efficiency indicators, statutory indicators, and insolvency information. The *National Committee for Quality Assurance (NCQA)* is responsible for carrying HEDIS forward. A second version of the reporting system, HEDIS 2.0, was released in 1993.

Health Promotion

See also:
Wellness;
Wellness Program

Refers to any type of community, employer-based, or individual program that encourages behavioral and environmental changes, eliminates risk hazards, and raises a person's awareness of physical fitness and good health. Many businesses are instituting health promotion programs as an effective way to reduce employee health care costs.

Health Resources and Services Administration (HRSA)

See also:
Maternal and Infant Care Program (MIC); National Practitioner Data Bank (NPDB)

A federal agency of the U.S. Public Health Service within the Department of Health and Human Services (HHS) responsible for developing primary health care services and resources, protecting and improving the health of mothers, infants, and children, improving access to care for the medically underserved and those with special needs, and maintaining a high quality of health care nationally. The HRSA has five major operating components: Office of the Administrator; Bureau of Health Professions, which administers the *National Practitioner Data Bank (NPDB)*; Bureau of Health Resources Development; Bureau of Primary Health Care; Maternal & Child Health Bureau.
Address: HRSA, 5600 Fishers Lane, Room 14-45, Parklawn Bldg., Rockville, MD 20857
Phone: (301) 443-2086; Fax: (301) 443-1989

H

Health Risk Appraisal

See also:
Exclusions; Health Status

A type of survey used by insurers, managed care plans, and employers to determine the likelihood of an insured person or plan member experiencing illness, injury or death in the future. The health risk appraisal also may be used to identify *exclusions* from coverage or to deny coverage.

Health Services Agreement (HSA)

See also:
Benefit(s) Package

A detailed description of health care procedures and benefits available for each employee enrolled in an employer-sponsored group health plan. The health services agreement is used as the basis of discussion and/or explanation between the employer and the health plan regarding enrollment, eligibility limitations, benefits, premiums, etc.

Health Standards Board (HSB)

See also:
Jackson Hole Group (JHG);
Managed Competition

One of three proposed private sector organizations which would be created under the *managed competition* model for health care reform developed by the *Jackson Hole Group*. The HSB would assess medical technologies and variations in medical practice, and also advise on effective services. The HSB would be sponsored by insurance, employer, consumer and provider groups.

Health Status

See also:
Quality Indicator;
Outcomes Measurement

Refers to the patient's state of health, which is usually assessed in terms of absence of disease or disability. Health status also may be assessed by the presence or absence of personal health habits which affect long term health (e.g., smoking), by family history, by occupational status, or some combination of these. Health status is considered a measure of outcome by organizations seeking to identify indicators of health care quality.

Healthcare Provider Networks Section of the AHA (HPNS)

See also:
Society for Healthcare Planning and Marketing (SHPM)

A special membership subgroup of the American Hospital Association's *Society for Healthcare Planning and Marketing (SHPM)*, formed in 1992 for health care professionals dealing with managed care issues. HPNS addresses policies and critical issues of managed care. HPNS also serves as an information clearinghouse on managed care services and activities, and encourages the exchange of information vital to the successful advancement of managed care programs.
Address: HPNS, 840 N. Lake Shore Drive,
Chicago, IL 60611
Phone: (312) 280-6086; Fax: (312) 280-6252

H

Hill Burton Act

See also:
State Health Planning and Development Agency (SHPDA)

Federal legislation passed in 1946 and amended frequently over the years, which provides federal support for construction and modernization of hospitals and other health care facilities. It is administered by each *state's health planning and development agency.* Also known as the "Hospital Survey and Construction Act of 1946."

HMO Act

See also:
Dual Choice;
Federally Qualified HMO (FQHMO)

A 1973 federal law which requires employers that are not self-insured, have more than 25 employees, and provide health coverage to offer a *federally qualified HMO (FQHMO)* to employees, whether as the only health benefit plan or in addition to other plans. Originally, the HMO Act specified minimum benefits and also provided seed money to establish different types of HMOs. Over time, however, the Act has been substantially amended to be less rigid in requirements.

HMO Group, The

See also:
Federally Qualified HMO;
Health Plan Employer Data & Information Set (HEDIS)

A national alliance of 21 non-profit, federally qualified, independent group and staff model HMOs, formed in 1984 for the purpose of defining and strengthening the HMOs' quality and performance. The HMO Group offers members on-site reviews to assure delivery of quality care and service, customer satisfaction surveys, a central resource for information sharing on operational and product concerns, publications, educational conferences, and seminars. The HMO Group participated in the development of the *Health Plan Employer Data and Information Set (HEDIS),* a standardized data collection and reporting system for assuring purchasers of the quality of HMO services.
Address: The HMO Group, 100 Albany St., Suite 230, New Brunswick, NJ 08901
Phone: (908) 220-1388; Fax: (908) 220-0298

Hold-Harmless Clause

See also:
No Balance Billing Clause

A contractual clause often found in managed care contracts between a payer and a provider. Under the hold-harmless clause, the provider agrees not to sue or make any claims against a plan member for covered services even if the plan becomes insolvent or fails to meet its financial obligations. Often used as a synonym for *no balance billing clause.*

Home Health Care

See also:
Home Healthcare Agency (HHA);
Hospice Care

Medical care provided by trained personnel in the patient's home for patients who do not need the more extensive treatment provided by a hospital, skilled nursing facility, or extended care facility, or for patients who are not capable of going to a medical facility for outpatient care. Often, home health care is preferred in the interests of the ease and comfort of the patient. Services include *hospice care*, infusion therapy, specialized pediatric and maternal/child programs, enterostomal therapy, physical, speech, and occupational therapy, and other specialized services. Many managed care plans use home health care when appropriate as a cost-containment technique. Services usually are provided by a *home healthcare agency.*

H

Home Healthcare Agency (HHA)

See also:
Home Health Care

An agency or organization that is licensed, certified, or otherwise authorized according to state and federal laws to provide skilled nursing and other therapeutic services to patients in their homes when the patients do not need or are not able to go to a health care facility for outpatient care. HHAs are governed by policies established by a professional group associated with the agency, which must include at least one physician and registered nurse. Generally, complete medical records must be maintained on each patient, and the HHA must have a full-time administrator.

Homemaker Service

An agency which provides the services of trained homemakers for individuals needing assistance in the home during illness or in situations where the parent or guardian is absent from the home.

Homeopathic

See also:
Alternative Therapies

A system of medicine whereby the cure of disease is believed to be affected by minute doses of drugs that produce the same symptoms in a healthy person as are present in the disease for which the drugs are administered. This is thought to stimulate physiological defenses against the signs and symptoms of the disease. Homeopathy as a formal system of medicine is no longer practiced in the United States. However, it may be informally practiced as an *alternative therapy*.

Horizontal Integration (HI)

See also:
Hospital Alliance;
Vertical Integration

A competitive strategy used by some hospitals to control the geographical distribution of health care services. Two common horizontal integration models are *hospital alliances* and holding companies. In an alliance, two or more hospitals form an alliance for the purpose of managed care contracting, to develop joint clinical services or regional centers of excellence, or to pursue business opportunities that could not be suppported by the hospitals individually. Hospitals in the alliance typically retain their individual autonomy, but may share information and services and do joint planning. In the holding company model, several hospitals form a separate parent company with its own board. The holding company has collective control of the participating hospitals' assets, and decisions are made by the board. The holding company model enables hospitals to consolidate services in order to reduce duplication, streamline decision making, and form and allocate capital.

Hospice Care
See also:
Continuum of Care;
Home Health Care;
Terminally Ill

An organized program that provides palliative and supportive care for *terminally ill* patients either at home or in a hospice (a type of facility specifically for terminally ill patients) rather than in a hospital or other type of acute care facility. Hospice care is provided by an interdisciplinary team of professionals and volunteers in a variety of settings, both inpatient and at home. Hospice care generally includes: skilled nursing services, medical and social services, psychological and dietary counseling, and also bereavement counseling for the family. Hospice care differs from *home health care* in that hospice services are provided to both the patient and the family, and usually increase with the patient's declining health, whereas home health services are provided only to the patient and tend to move from more frequent to less frequent visits as the patient recovers. Costs for hospice care are usually covered by Medicare, Medicaid, and most private insurance plans.

H

Hospital Affiliation
See also:
Health Services;
Participating Provider

A contractual agreement between a managed care plan and one or more hospitals whereby the hospital(s) provide the inpatient *health services* covered by the health plan. Hospital affiliation may also refer to a physician's staff privileges at a hospital.

Hospital Alliance
See also:
Horizontal Integration (HI);
Voluntary Hospital

A group of *voluntary hospitals* (i.e., not-for-profit) which join together to reduce costs and achieve economies of scale by sharing common services and developing group purchasing programs. Hospital alliances are usually formed to improve competitive positions over other provider institutions and multihospital systems. An example is Voluntary Hospitals of America, Inc., which currently is the largest not-gor-profit hospital alliance in the nation.

Hospital Days

See: **Bed Days** and **Length of Stay (LOS)**

Hospital-Physician Alliance (HPA)

See also:
Integrated Delivery System (IDS); Management Service Organization (MSO); Physician-Hospital Organization (PHO); Safe Harbor Regulations

A partnership between a hospital and some or all of its staff physicians. There are many different types of hospital-physician alliances, ranging from an informal sharing of expertise, in which the hospital provides assistance in office staff training, marketing, educational programs, etc., to a more structured arrangement, involving computer networking, assistance with physician recruitment, and practice development. Examples of formal business structures include: *physician-hospital organizations (PHO)* for managed care contracting, *management service organizations (MSO)* for practice management, and *integrated delivery systems (IDS)* for joint development of a broad range of clinical services (e.g., ambulatory care, home health care).

Hybrid HMO

See also:
Mixed Model Managed Care Plan

A type of HMO which includes service features of indemnity insurance, such as coinsurance, deductibles, experience rating, open panel of providers, in addition to the various utilization, cost, and access controls and structures of prepaid HMO-type health plans. Sometimes called a *mixed model managed care plan.*

I

Iatrogenic Disease

See also:
Complication

Any disease-related injury or *complication* brought on by the process of medical testing, clinical procedures, surgery, medication, or non-optimal nursing care. Examples of medically induced disease include: allergic reactions to medications, stress ulcers, bedsores, postoperative infections, etc. Also called *medically induced disease.*

In-Area Services

See also:
Out-of-Area Services; Service Area

Covered health care services received by a plan member from a participating provider within the managed care plan's authorized geographical *service area.*

In-Network Services

See also:
Participating Provider; Out-of-Network Services

Covered health care services received by a plan member from a *participating provider* of the health plan. (Contrast with *out-of-network services.*)

Incentive Plan

See also:
Cost-Sharing Techniques; Non-Participatory Provider (NonPar); Preferred Provider

An employee health benefit plan which offers employees a financial incentive to use *preferred providers.* For example, the deductible may be reduced, coinsurance may be raised to a higher percentage, the out-of-pocket limit may be lowered, or any combination of these, as an incentive for using a preferred provider. If an employee uses a *non-participatory provider (nonpar),* the health benefits remain at the current level with no financial incentive. The incentive plan approach aims to lower the employer's health care costs by offering employees greater benefits with little or no increase in costs to the employer.

Incontestable Clause

See also:
Non-Cancelable Guaranteed Renewable Policy

An optional clause in some health insurance contracts which states that the insurer may not contest the validity of the contract after it has been in force for two (sometimes three) years. An incontestable clause sometimes is used in *non-cancelable guaranteed renewable policies.*

Incurred But Not Reported (IBNR)

See also:
Claim Lag Studies

A financial calculation used by health plans to identify the costs associated with a medical service which has been provided to a plan member but has not yet been submitted as a claim. Health plans must maintain and record IBNR reserves to account for estimated liability based on studies of prior lags in claim submission (see *claim lag studies*). Sometimes called *incurred but unreported claims (IUC).*

Incurred Claims

See also:
Claims Reserve

An accounting term which describes an insurance carrier's total liability for a specified period, usually a policy year (called the "experience period"). *Incurred claims* equal all claims paid during the policy year, plus the *claims reserve* as of the end of the policy year, minus the corresponding claims reserve as of year-beginning. The difference between the year-end and the year-beginning claims reserves is called the "increase in reserves." This amount is added to the paid claims to produce the incurred claims. Due to the time lag between the dates of service and claim payments, such adjustments must be made to any claims data in order to determine incurred claims.

Incurred Claims Loss Ratio (ICLR)

See also:
Incurred Claims;
Loss Ratio

A financial indicator used by health plans to compare total claims liability to the amount of premium paid during a specified period. The ICLR is derived by dividing *incurred claims* by premiums.

Indemnity Insurance See: **Fee-for-Service Insurance**

Independent Practice Association (IPA)

See also:
Capitaiton;
IPA Model HMO

A group of physicians who have formed an association as a separate legal entity for the purpose of managed care contracting to provide services in their own offices. IPA members are compensated on a *capitation* basis for contracts with *IPA model HMOs* or a fee-for-service basis for medical services provided to members of other types of managed care plans. Referrals typically are made to specialists within the IPA. IPA members remain individual practitioners, retain their separate officies, continue to see their non-managed care patients, and also retain their ability to contract directly with managed care plans. A key advantage of the IPA arrangement is that it helps its members achieve some of the negotiating benefits of belonging to a group practice.

Indicator

See also:
Quality Indicator

A measurable aspect of the health care delivery process which signifies whether or not the appropriate clinical interventions were provided to the patient during the course of treatment. Selected indicators, such as clinical outcome (e.g., mortality and morbidity), health status, length of stay, readmission rate, patient satisfaction, etc., are considered to be indicators of the quality of care. However, no universally recognized set of indicators has been accepted as the industry standard for quality of care.

Individual Case Management

See also:
Case Management;
Utilization Management (UM)

A *utilization management* (*UM*) technique whereby an individual case (usually a high-cost case) is managed by a dedicated team of UM professionals in order to find the most appropriate and cost-effective care, even if it involves paying for services not routinely covered by the health plan. For example, a managed care plan may build a wheelchair ramp or install air conditioning in a patient's home so that the patient can go home from the hospital earlier and receive any necessary further treatment in a less costly outpatient setting.

Individual Case Management Association (ICMA)

See also:
Case Manager (CM)

A professional organization which represents independently practicing *case managers (CM)* who contract with managed care organizations, self-funded employers, and insurers to provide CM services in a specific geographical area. ICMA offers members educational programs, including seminars and a national conference, a national databank of CMs and other medical and disability management professionals, networking opportunities, publications (CM Trends, The Case Manager, ICMA Directory), and other personal training and resource materials. ICMA initiated a national CM certification program in 1991, which now is administered by the Certified Insurance Rehabilitation Specialists Commission.
Address: ICMA, 10809 Executive Center Drive
Suite 105, Little Rock, AR 72211-6020
Phone: (501) 227-5553; Fax: (501) 227-8362

I

Industry Adjustment Factor (IAF)

See also:
Community Rating by Class (CRC)

A weighting factor used by some HMOs that use *community rating by class (CRC)* methodology to adjust a group's premium rates in an effort to predict and account for that group's expected level of health care utilization. IAFs frequently are used as a means for managed care plans to give discounts to their commercial accounts.

Inflow

See also:
Outflow;
Service Area

The number of people who are not residents of a defined *service area* but who obtain care from providers in the area. Inflow information is obtained from an analysis of the origins of patients that use providers in the defined service area. For example, in forecasting use of new inpatient services, inflow is typically presented as a percentage of total admissions. Thus, if 20% of all patients that use local hospitals reside in other areas, the inflow is 20%.

Injury

See also:
Injury Independent of All Other Means

Refers to any physiological damage other than sickness, including all related conditions and recurrent symptoms.

Injury Independent of All Other Means

See also:
Injury

An injury resulting from an accident, provided that the accident was not caused by an illness.

Inpatient (IP)

See also:
Inpatient Services; Outpatient (OP)

A person who is admitted to a hospital for medical care, is assigned a bed designated for routine, special, psychiatric, or rehabilitation care, and occupies the bed overnight. The antonym is *outpatient (OP)*.

Inpatient Services

See also:
Inpatient (IP)

Medical services provided in a hospital to a plan member who has been admitted and occupies a hospital bed in order to receive care. Inpatient services include room, board, general nursing care, diagnostic treatment, and other hospital-based health services.

Insurable Risk

See also:
Uninsurable Risk

Refers to the conditions that make a health risk insurable. Insurable risk generally includes the following conditions: 1) the peril that is insured against must produce a definite loss not under the control of the insured; 2) there must be a large number of homogeneous exposures which are subject to the same perils; 3) the loss must be quantifiable and the cost of insuring it must be economically feasible; 4) the peril must be unlikely to affect all the insured persons simultaneously; and 5) the loss produced by the risk must be definite and have a potential to be financially serious. (Contrast with *uninsurable risk*.)

Insuring Clause

A clause in a health insurance contract which sets forth the type of loss being covered by the policy and also the parties to the insurance contract.

Integrated Deductible

See also:
Comprehensive Major Medical Insurance; Corridor Deductible; Deductible

Refers to the greater of two *deductible* amounts, a fixed dollar amount and the amount of basic medical benefits that are paid in a *comprehensive major medical insurance* plan. Once this amount of out-of- pocket expense (i.e., the integrated deductible) is reached, supplemental major benefits are then payable by the insurance carrier. Sometimes called *corridor deductible.*

Integrated Delivery System (IDS)

See also:
Community Care Network; Continuum of Care

A local or regional health care network which provides a full range of services for all aspects of health care (i.e., a *continuum of care*) for patients in a defined geographical area. The services may include wellness programs, preventive care, ambulatory clinics, out-patient diagnostic and laboratory services, emergency care, general hospital services, rehabilitation, long-term care, congregate living, psychiatric care, home health and hospice care. Typically, an IDS establishes strategic alliances and contractual relationships with other providers for those services not provided directly by the IDS. Presumably, because the IDS offers many alternatives to inpatient care, it is better able to provide and coordinate high quality, cost-effective care, and also assume the financial risk involved in fixed-rate (capitated) contracts. Sometimes called a *community care network* or an *organized system of care (OSC).*

Intensive Care Unit (ICU)

See also:
Coronary Care Unit (CCU)

A distinctive care unit within a hospital which has specialized equipment and staff who provide a higher, more intense level of care and surveillance to patients needing more than the standard level of hospital care. ICU patients are under constant personal observation by a specially trained nurse who has all necessary lifesaving equipment, drugs and supplies immediately available.

Interdisciplinary Audit

See also:
Intradisciplinary Audit

A type of evaluation of a patient's medical care in which two or more health care professionals from different disciplines develop criteria applicable to several disciplines and analyze medical records that vary from their criteria. The purpose of an interdisciplinary audit is to assess quality for the respective types of care provided.

Intermediate Care Facility (ICF)

A health care facility which provides an intermediate level of care to patients who require care above the level of room and board, but not the level of care and treatment that a hospital or skilled nursing facility (SNF) is designed to provide. Sometimes called a *transitional care facility*.

Intermediate Outcome

See also:
Outcomes

The anticipated patient status relative to a specific treatment plan at a particular point in time during the treatment process.

Internal Medicine

See also:
Gatekeeper;
Primary Care Physician (PCP)

The field of medicine which deals primarily with diseases of the internal organs and with services usually provided by physicians whose specialty is internal medicine. An internal medicine specialist (also called an internist) is considered a *primary care physician (PCP)* by most managed care plans, and as such, may serve as a *gatekeeper* for plan members seeking medical care.

International Classification of Disease, 9th Edition (ICD-9)

See also:
Diagnosis-Related Group (DRG)

A standardized coding system consisting of a listing of diagnoses and associated identification codes. The ICD-9 coding system is used by physicians for reporting diagnoses of covered persons on claims. The coding and terminology provide a uniform language, which accurately designates primary and secondary diagnoses and also ensures reliable, consistent communication on claim forms. ICD-9 codes are required on all Medicare claim forms and Medicare itemized billing statements.

International Foundation of Employee Benefit Plans (IFEBP)

An educational association in the employee benefits field which offers its members information services, publications, educational programs, on-line benefits database, research publications, certification program, and a student "I.F. Interns" program. Total membership in 1993 consisted of 34,000 individuals representing more than 7,500 trust funds, public employee funds, corporations, and professional firms throughout the U.S. and Canada.
Address: IFEBP, 18700 W. Bluemound Road,
P.O. Box 69, Brookfield, WI 53008-0069
Phone: (414) 786-6700; Fax: (414) 786-2990

I

International Subacute Healthcare Association (ISHA)

See also:
Intermediate Care Facility (ICF); Subacute Care

A trade association representing the interests of subacute and transitional providers and practitioners. ISHA is developing industry standards and guidelines to help payors, health care personnel, and the public identify quality subacute and transitional care providers. Membership services include: educational seminars and materials, networking opportunities, a resource library, monthly newsletter, and legislative and regulatory representation regarding policies that impact subacute and transitional care providers.
Address: ISHA, 4040 W. 70th Street,
Minneapolis, MN 55435
Phone: (612) 926-1773; Fax: (612) 926-1624

InterStudy

See also:
Health Outcomes Institute (HOI); Jackson Hole Group (JHG); Outcomes Management System (OMS); Outcomes Research

A research organization specializing in managed care research, particularly of HMOs. InterStudy maintains a database on HMO enrollment, characteristics, and qualification status. Its publications include the Competitive Edge, an HMO directory, and a series of monographs on outcomes research. InterStudy developed a methodology for measuring health care outcomes, called the *Outcomes Management System (OMS),* which was turned over to *Health Outcomes Institute*, an *outcomes research* organization, in February, 1993. In July, 1993, InterStudy was acquired by Decision Resources, a health care publishing and consulting firm in Waltham, MA.
Address: InterStudy, 2901 Metro Drive, Suite 400, Bloomington, MN 55331
Phone: (612) 858-9291; Fax: (612) 854-5698

Intradisciplinary Audit

See also:
Interdisciplinary Audit

A type of retrospective evaluation study of a patient's medical care in which several health care professionals representing a single discipline develop criteria and analyze medical records that have variations from pre-established criteria. The intradisciplinary audit is limited to those aspects of the patient's care that fall into the area of responsibility of intradisciplinary team members. Sometimes called *monodisciplinary audit.*

IPA Model HMO

See also:
Independent Practice Association (IPA); Open Panel

An *open panel* type of HMO which contracts with an association of physicians, called an *independent practice association (IPA)*, to provide services to its members. The IPA is set up as a separate legal entity for contracting purposes. Physician members remain independent practitioners, maintain their own offices, medical records and office staff, and continue to see their non-HMO patients. An IPA Model HMO compensates the IPA on a physician capitation basis. The IPA in turn compensates its members on either a fee-for-service basis or a combination of fee-for-service and "primary care capitation" (i.e., primary care physicians are paid on a capitated basis and specialists are paid on a fee schedule or *usual, customary, and reasonable* basis). Typically, the IPA withholds a portion of payments for risk-sharing and incentive purposes.

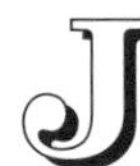

Jackson Hole Group (JHG)

See also:
InterStudy; Managed Competition;

A non-profit organization which studies and lobbies for health care reform. JHG, led by Dr. Paul Ellwood, founder of *InterStudy,* is advancing the *managed competition* model for national health care reform. In this model, large health insurance purchasing cooperatives would be created for small employers and individuals. Accountable health partnerships would act as both insurer and provider, and a national health board would develop and oversee a standard benefits package.

Joint Commission on Accreditation of Healthcare Organizations (JCAHO)

See also:
Accreditation;
Integrated Delivery System (IDS)

A private, non-profit organization which functions as the main accrediting body for hospitals and other provider facilities. JCAHO's seeks to improve health care quality by publishing national standards, surveying facilities on request, and awarding accreditation to those that demonstrate compliance with the standards. JCAHO accreditation is voluntary, but is a required for participation in Medicare. JCAHO is now developing accreditation standards applicable specifically to health care networks, which are being published in 1994. Relevant performance measures will be developed, tested, and introduced over the next two years.
Address: JCAHO, One Renaissance Blvd., Oakbrook Terrace, IL 60181
Phone: (708) 916-5800; Fax: (708) 916-5644

Joint Powers Authority (JPA)

See also:
Health Insurance Purchasing Cooperative (HIPC);
Managed Competition

A type of health insurance purchasing cooperative for school districts, whereby several different school districts form into one larger group for the purpose of soliciting and purchasing health care coverage on a more cost-effective basis than direct purchases of traditionally insured plans by individual school districts. JPAs are similar in many respects to the *health insurance purchasing cooperative (HIPC)* concept in the *managed competition* model for national health care reform.

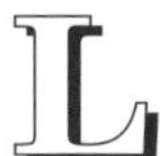

Lapse

See also:
Reinstatement
Renewal

Cancellation of a health insurance policy when a policyholder fails to pay the premium within the time required.

Large Case Management (LCM)

See: **Case Management**

Large Claim Pooling

See also:
Claims Pooling;
Pooling

In experience rating, refers to the practice of separating out large claim amounts over a certain defined level, or "pooling point" ($30,000, for example), and charging these amounts to a pool, which is funded by the pooled charges of all groups who share this defined *pooling* level. The purpose of large claim pooling is to help stabilize premium fluctuations, which tend to occur more often with smaller group sizes. Smaller groups generally have lower pooling points and larger groups tend to have higher pooling points.

Legal Reserve

See also:
Claim Reserves;
Loss Reserve

The minimum amount of money that an insurer must keep in reserve to meet future claims and obligations. The amount of the legal reserve is calculated under state insurance codes.

Legend Drug

See: **Prescription Drug**

Length of Stay (LOS)

See also:
Average Length of Stay (ALOS);
Bed Days;
Patient Day(s)

The number of days a patient is hospitalized as an inpatient for each episode of illness or injury. LOS can refer to the patient's total number of days of hospitalization per episode of care, or to the number of days in a particular unit or level of care. Sometimes called *discharge days* or *hospital days.*

License/Licensure

A permission granted to an individual or organization by a recognized authority to lawfully engage in a certain practice, occupation, or activity. License is usually granted on the basis of examination or proof of education rather than on measures of performance. A license is usually permanent; however, it may be conditioned on annual payment of a fee, proof of continuing education, or proof of competence. *Licensure* is the process by which a license is granted.

Licensed Practical Nurse (LPN)

See also:
Registered Nurse (RN).

A nurse who is licensed by the state to carry out specified nursing duties under the direction of a *registered nurse (RN).* LPNs have formal training in practical or vocational nursing educational programs but are not graduates of a formal diploma school. Also called *licensed vocational nurse (LVN).*

Licensed Vocational Nurse (LVN)

See: **Licensed Practical Nurse (LPN)**

L

Life Care at Home Program (LCAH)

See also:
Continuing Care Retirement Community (CCRC);
Long-Term Care (LTC)

A relatively new, low cost, guaranteed-access *long-term care* program for Medicaid recipients. The program offers many of the same benefits as a *continuing care retirement community (CCRC)* program, but allows the elderly to remain in their own homes instead of moving to a central campus. Generally, LCAH programs provide comprehensive coverage for both nursing home and home-based care by using a number of managed care and risk management techniques (e.g., case management) to control costs.

Life Expectancy

See also:
Mortality Rate

The length of time a person of a given age is expected to live. Life expectancy is a statistical average based on mortality tables showing *mortality rates* at each age. The life expectancy indicator does not seek to predict the life span of any particular individual.

Lifetime Disability Benefit

See also:
Total Disability

An insurance benefit designed to help replace income lost by the covered person as long as he/she is totally disabled, even for a lifetime.

Lifetime Reserve

See also:
Medicare

A non-renewable lifetime reserve of sixty days of hospitalization available to a *Medicare* beneficiary to draw on if the standard ninety covered days per benefit period are exhausted.

Limited Policy

A restricted benefits insurance contract which covers only certain specified diseases or accidents.

Line of Business (LOB)

Refers to a managed care plan that is set up as a separate business unit within another larger organization (e.g., life insurance company). For example, a large health insurance company may have an HMO, a PPO, and utilization management as individual "lines of business" in addition to its traditional indemnity insurance business. The LOB designation legally diffentiates the managed care plans from a free-standing company or one set up as a subsidiary. LOB also may refer to a unique product type, such as Medicaid, within a health plan.

Lives

In insurance, the number of individuals or employees in a particular group covered by a group health plan.

Long-Term Care (LTC)

See also:
Activities of Daily Living (ADL)

A type of care which includes broad-based health maintenance, personal care, and health care services to the chronically ill, disabled, or retarded. Health services may be provided on an inpatient basis, for example, in a rehabilitation facility, nursing home, mental hospital, or home for the retarded, or on an outpatient or at-home basis. The goal of LTC is to help people who need assistance with the *activities of daily living (ADL)* be as independent as possible. The focus of LTC is more on "caring" than on "curing."

Long-Term Disability Income Insurance

See also:
Lifetime Disability Benefit

A type of insurance issued to an employer or individual to provide a reasonable replacement of a portion of an employee's earned income lost through serious and prolonged illness or injury during the normal work career.

Loss Ratio

See also:
Incurred Claims Loss Ratio (ICLR);
Net Loss Ratio (NLR)

An indicator used by insurers as a way of measuring the amount of benefits returned to policyholders. The loss ratio compares an employer's actual claims experience to the premium paid. For example, a low loss ratio indicates a "good" claims experience for a given period, and also shows that the premium collected was more than required to fund the actual claims. A high loss ratio shows that claims exceeded the premium for the given time period.

Loss Reserve

See also:
Claim Reserves; Incurred But Not Reported (IBNR); Legal Reserve

An amount representing the estimated financial liability for unpaid insurance claims (losses) that have occurred as of a given date. The loss reserve includes losses *incurred but not reported (INBR)*, claims being adjusted, and amounts known to be payable in the future (e.g., long-term disability). A health plan's loss reserve appears as a line item on its financial statement. On an individual basis, a loss reserve represents an estimate of the total amount to be paid out on a particular claim.

Low Volume DRGs

See also:
Diagnosis-Related Group (DRG)

A special category in the *DRG* classification system for those DRGs having five or less patients in a hospital's base year.

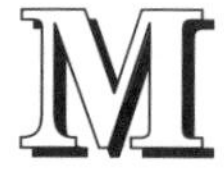

Magnetic Resonance Imaging (MRI)

See also:
Ancillary Services

A non-invasive diagnostic procedure of imaging soft tissues using a powerful magnet and radio waves to produce computer-processed images of the inner body. MRI is often used in the diagnosis of many diseases involving the head, spinal column, and certain joints. A relatively new MRI technique for detecting blockages in coronary arteries shows promise as a cost-effective replacement for conventional angiography, or "cardiac catherization." As a diagnostic *ancillary service,* MRI normally requires a physician referral and prior authorization from the managed care plan for full payment of benefits.

Mail Order Pharmacy A method of dispensing medication directly to the patient through the mail by means of a mail order drug distribution company. The pharmaceutical industry estimates that ninety million prescriptions are filled annually by mail order pharmacies at considerable cost savings to the purchasers. Mail order drug distributors can purchase drugs in larger volumes than retail or wholesale outlets and can therefore offer greatly reduced costs for prescriptions. Many employers that include a mail order option in their drug benefit programs give their employees financial incentives to use a mail order pharmacy when it is appropriate, especially for long-term drug therapy. Also called *mail service pharmacy*.

Maintenance of Benefits Plan (MOB)

See also:
Eligible Expenses

A type of Medicare supplement plan in which charges paid by Medicare are subtracted from the total *eligible expenses*. Health benefits of the normal plan, including deductibles, coinsurance, and any other plan provisions, are then applied to these remaining expenses. Only those eligible expenses not paid by Medicare are considered for reimbursement under an MOB plan. Also called an *eligible expense offset plan.*

Major Diagnostic Categories (MDC)

See also:
Diagnosis-Related Group (DRG)

A set of 23 broad classifications of diagnoses which are categorized primarily according to organ system. MDCs are the first step in identifying *diagnostic related groups (DRGs).*

Major Medical Insurance

See also:
Comprehensive Major Medical Insurance; Fee-for-Service Insurance

A traditional *fee-for-service insurance* plan which covers most medical expenses up to a high dollar amount (e.g., up to $250,000, or unlimited). Major medical insurance often includes an initial deductible and coinsurance, and reimburses the major portion of all charges for hospital, physician, private nurses, medical appliances, prescribed treatments, drugs, etc. The insured pays the remainder. Full reimbursement is often provided once the expenses paid by the insured reach a certain level. This type of insurance usually does not cover routine or preventive care, or catastrophic types of illness.

Malpractice

See also:
Defensive Medicine; Malpractice Insurance

Refers to professional misconduct, dereliction from professional duty, or lack of ordinary skill in the performance of a professional act, which results in death, injury, loss, or damage to the patient. A practitioner is liable for damages or injuries caused by malpractice. However, malpractice requires that the patient prove that the injury was negligently caused.

Malpractice Insurance

See also:
Professional Liability Insurance (PLI)

Insurance against the financial liability from a lawsuit resulting from injury to a patient caused by alleged negligence in treating the patient. Also known as *professional liability insurance (PLI).*

Managed Care

See also:
Alternative Delivery Systems (ADS);
Coordinated Care;
Managed Care Plan (MCP)

A system of managing and financing health care delivery to ensure that services provided to managed care plan members are necessary, efficiently provided, and appropriately priced. Through a variety of techniques, such as preadmission certification, concurrent review, financial incentives or penalties, managed care attempts to control access to provider sites where services are received, contain costs, manage utilization of services and resources, and ensure favorable patient outcomes. The term covers a broad spectrum of arrangements for health care delivery and financing, including managed indemnity plans (MIP), health maintenance organizations (HMO), preferred provider organizations (PPO), point-of-service plans (POS), as well as direct contracting arrangements between employers and providers. Sometimes called *alternative delivery systems (ADS)* or *coordinated care.*

Managed Care Network

See also:
Managed Care Plan (MCP);
Network Adequacy;
Provider Panel

A regional or national organization of providers which is owned by a commercial insurance company or other sponsor (e.g., a *managed care plan)* and offered to employers and other groups or organizations as either an alternative to or a total replacement for traditional indemnity health insurance.

Managed Care Organization (MCO)

See also:
Managed Care Plan (MCP)

A generic term referring to a managed care plan or a managed care company, such as an HMO, PPO, or exclusive provider organization (EPO). Often, the term is used interchangeably with *managed care plan.*

Managed Care Plan (MCP)

See also:
Managed Care;
Managed Care Network;
Provider Panel

A type of group health plan designed to provide appropriate, efficient, and cost-effective health services to enrollees through contractual arrangements with selected providers. MCPs typically include formal programs of quality assurance and utilization review, and also financial incentives for enrollees to use providers associated with the plan. In the past, the term usually was associated with HMOs, but now MCP includes many other plan types, such as preferred provider organizations (PPO), managed indemnity plans (MIP), exclusive provider organizations (EPO), point-of-service plans (POS). Also, direct contracting arrangements between employers and providers may be considered a type of MCP.

Managed Choice

See also:
Point-of-Service Plan (POS);
Self-Referral

A type of managed care plan which combines elements of managed care, such as restricted provider choice, and traditional indemnity insurance with no restrictions on provider selection. For example, a managed choice plan may provide HMO-type benefits for authorized services along with an option to *self-refer* at a significantly lower benefit level. Each plan member usually selects a primary care physician as a gatekeeper, who serves as the member's health care "manager." Also called *open-ended HMO*, *swing-out HMO,* and *point-of-service plan (POS).*

Managed Competition

See also:
American Health Security Act of 1993 (AHSA);
Health Insurance Purchasing Cooperative (HIPC);
Jackson Hole Group (JHG);
Managed Care Organization (MCO)

A model for national health care reform developed by the *Jackson Hole Group*. Managed competition calls for partnerships between providers and insurers. Large purchasing groups, called *health insurance purchasing cooperatives (HIPCs)*, would pool the purchasing power of many consumers to buy a standard benefits package from qualified *managed care organizations*. Employers would no longer arrange health care coverage for their employees. Instead, both employers and employees would contribute to a public fund that would funnel revenue to the HIPCs. The idea is to force providers to compete on the basis of price and quality. The MCOs would serve as "sponsors," dividing providers into economic groups for competitive contracting. Many features of the managed competition model have been incorporated in President Clinton's proposal for national health care reform, called the *American Health Security Act of 1993.*

M

Managed Fee-for-Service Insurance

See: **Managed Indemnity Plan (MIP)**

Managed Health Care Association (MHCA)

See also:
Health Plan Employer Data and Information Set (HEDIS); Outcomes Management System (OMS)

A national trade organization representing over 120 large employers which have implemented or are considering managed care programs. MHCA provides a forum for exchange of ideas and experiences on how to manage health care programs for better results, with an emphasis on measuring quality, service levels, cost performance, and employee and patient satisfaction. MHCA fosters education and training for benefits and health care management professionals through annual national meetings, dissemination of information on public policy and innovative managed care projects, and publications. MHCA also is involved in projects for standardizing outcomes and managed care data measures, such as the *Outcomes Management System (OMS)* project and the *Health Plan Employer Data and Information Set (HEDIS)* for measuring the value of managed care to employers.
Address: MHCA, 1225 Eye St., NW, Suite 300, Washington DC 20005
Phone: (202) 371-8232; Fax: (202) 842-0621

M

Managed Indemnity Plan (MIP)

See also:
Fee-for-Service Insurance (FFS); Managed Care Plan (MCP)

An indemnity health insurance plan that incorporates some managed care techniques, like required second surgical opinion, preadmisssion certification, and concurrent utilization review, to control costs and ensure the quality of services provided to plan members. Unlike *managed care plans*, MIPs offer members the same latitude in choosing providers as traditional, "unmanaged" fee-for-service insurance. Sometimes called *managed fee-for-service insurance.*

Management Information System (MIS)

See also:
Community Health Information System (CHMIS);
Employee Benefits Information System (EBIS)

Integrated computer hardware and software systems used by many managed care organizations (MCO) and self-insured employers for administering their health plans. Managed care applications include: automated claims processing, clinical record-keeping, encounter processing, utilization review, clinical outcomes tracking, and physician resource utilization studies. Some MCOs use MIS as a strategic tool to demonstrate delivery of high quality, cost-effective care in response to a growing demand for utilization data by employers.

Management Service Organization (MSO)

See also:
Multispecialty Group (MSG)

An organization formed by one or more physician group practices to manage their medical practices. Typically, the MSO furnishes sites, facilities, equipment, administrative services, and personnel, allowing the physicians to concentrate on practicing medicine. A key advantage for physicians is that they can continue to own and operate all clinical aspects of their practices, including charts and patients, but overhead is reduced through economies of scale. Also, an MSO is easier and faster to form than a *multispecialty group*. Some hospitals are developing MSOs in partnership with staff physicians, especially primary care physicians, to help their medical staff maintain autonomy and protect them against income erosion. Also called *Medical Service Organization.*

Mandated Benefits

See also:
ERISA;
Mandated Providers

Certain health care benefits required under federal or state law to be provided or made available to policy holders and eligible dependents by managed care organizations and insurance carriers. Usually mandated benefits are above and beyond routine insurance-type benefits. Some examples are: in-vitro fertilization, chiropractic services, a defined number of days of inpatient mental health or substance abuse treatment, etc. Currently, only self-funded plans are exempt from mandated benefits under *ERISA*.

Mandated Providers

See also:
Mandated Benefits

Providers of specialty health care services whose licensed services must, under state or federal law, be included in coverage offered by a health plan. Depending on state laws, mandated providers might be psychologists, optometrists, podiatrists, chiropractors, etc.

Manual Rate

See also:
Age/Sex Rates (ASR); Rating Process

A premium rate developed for a group health plan using the insurance carrier's standard rate tables, or "rate manual." The manual rate (i.e., derived from the rate manual) usually is based on the health plan's average claims data and then adjusted for group- specific variations in demographics, industry factors, or benefits. (An insurance carrier's standard rate tables are normally referred to as its *rate manual* or *underwriting manual.*)

Market Area

See also:
Catchment Area; Market Share; Service Area

Refers to a targeted geographical area or the areas of greatest market potential for managed care plan sales. Managed care organizations typically refer to their market areas when determining sales and marketing strategies for their managed care products. Often, the market area is larger than the managed care plan's defined *catchment area,* particularly when the plan is seeking to expand into new markets. Sometimes called *service area.*

Market Share

See also:
Market Area;
Utilization

A *utilization* index used in strategic planning and marketing to assess the proportion of an organization's business in a defined *market area* or for forecasting market demand. Market share may be determined for total existing business, specific lines of business, or specific services. For example, a hospital calculates its market share by dividing its patient volume (admissions) in a specified market area for a given period of time by the total number of admissions for all providers (or main competitors) for the defined *market area* and given time period.

Master Group Contract

See also:
Certificate of Coverage (COC);
Group Contract

A legally binding group health agreement between an employer (as the "enrolling unit") and an insurance carrier, which sets forth in detail the rights and obligations of the employer, the covered person(s), and the insurer, as well as the terms and conditions of the coverage provided under the contract. The terms and conditions of coverage also are described in the *certificate of coverage (COC),* which is provided by the plan to covered employees.

Maternal and Infant Care (MIC)

See also:
Health Resources and Services Administration (HRSA)

A federally funded program administered by the states for services to young, high-risk mothers and their infants during prenatal and perinatal periods.

Maximum Allowable Cost (MAC)

See also:
Drug Formulary

The maximum amount that a vendor may charge health care purchasers for products or services. Usually the term is used in reference to negotiated charges for selected drugs in a *drug formulary* in managed care contracting with pharmacies. Typically, a managed care plan or other health care purchaser develops a MAC list of prescription medications that will be covered at a generic drug level. The MAC list is distributed to participating pharmacies and is subject to periodic review and modifications by the plan. The federal government uses a MAC program to limit reimbursement for prescription drugs for Medicare and Medicaid beneficiaries. In these programs, the MAC is the lowest unit price at which a drug that is available from several sources can be purchased on a national basis and without significant inconvenience to beneficiaries.

Maximum Allowable Payment (MAP)

The maximum amount that a health plan will pay toward the cost of services incurred by an individual or family in a specified period, usually a calendar year. Also called *maximum benefit.*

Maximum Benefit

See: **Maximum Allowable Payment (MAP)**

Maximum Length of Stay (MaxLOS)

See also:
Average Length of Stay (ALOS);
Length of Stay (LOS)

A utilization management tool used by managed care plans to control hospital *length of stay (LOS)*. Plans that use a MaxLOS assign the LOS on the basis of the admission diagnosis and the *average length of stay (ALOS)* for that diagnosis, and will not authorize any additional days for payment. MaxLOS designations vary by geographical regions. Depending on the plan, exceeding the MaxLOS may result in denial of payment for services rendered after the MaxLOS has been reached or a reduction in payment by a percentage amount.

Maximum Out-of-Pocket Expense

See also:
Out-of-Pocket Payments (OOP)

Refers to the maximum amount that the insured will have to pay in deductibles and coinsurance before the health plan pays 100% for covered benefits. The primary purpose of the maximum out-of-pocket expense is to place a cap on catastrophic costs incurred by plan members.

Measurable

See also:
Indicator

The characteristic of being objectively quantifiable or assessable using standard measuring devices or methodologies.

Medicaid

See also:
Recipient;
Title XIX

A federal public assistance program administered and operated by participating state and territorial governments. Medicaid provides medical benefits to eligible low income persons (called *recipients*) needing health care regardless of age. Under *Title XIX* of the Social Security Act, effective January 1, 1966, the states receive federal matching grants to cover the costs of the program. Certain minimal services must be included to receive federal matching funds. However, the states may optionally include any additional services at state expense. Also known as *Title XIX*.

Medical Assistant (MA)

See: **Allied Health Professional**

Medical Care Evaluation (MCE)

See also:
Peer Review Organization (PRO)

A retrospective review study involving in-depth assessments of the quality of both the delivery of care and the organization of health care services. The purpose of MCE studies is to ensure that health care services are appropriate to the patients' needs and of optimal quality, and that the health care organization supports the timely provision of quality care. Medicare and Medicaid programs require hospital utilization review committees to have at least one MCE study in progress at all times. MCE studies are also required by *Peer Review Organization (PRO)* programs.

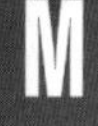

Medical Case Management (MCM)

See: **Case Management**

Medical Expense Reimbursement Plan (MERP)

See also:
Contributory Plan; Non-Contributory Plan

A type of employer-sponsored health plan in which the employer pays its employees' out-of-pocket medical expenses, as opposed to a *contributory plan* in which employees share in the cost of the premiums. Sometimes called a *non-contributory plan.*

Medical Foundation

See: **Foundation for Medical Care (FMC)**

Medical Group Management Association (MGMA)

See also:
Group Practice

A trade organization representing physicians, administrators, CEOs, office managers and other professionals involved in medical *group practices.* MGMA provides its members networking, professional development, and educational opportunities through special interest Assemblies, Alliances, and Societies, (e.g., the American College of Medical Group Administrators), and through seminars and an annual national conference. A Library Resource Center provides information on relevant legislative and regulatory activities, and consulting assistance in identifying and solving management problems. Technical support and advice for improving health care delivery and administrative processes of members' group practices is offered though its Center for Research in Ambulatory Care Administration. MGMA publishes the bimonthly MGM Journal, a monthly newspaper (MGM Update), a membership directory, and other subscription publications.
Address: MGMA, 104 Inverness Terrace East, Englewood, CO 80112-5306
Phone: (303) 799-1111; Fax: (303) 643-4427

Medical Loss Ratio (MLR)

See also:
Loss Ratio;
Net Loss Ratio

An index which compares the costs of delivering health benefits with the revenues received by the plan. The MLR is calculated by dividing the total medical expenses by the total revenue. Insurance companies often have an MLR of 96% or more. Well-managed HMOs may have MLRs of 75% to 85%.

Medical Negligence

See also:
Malpractice

Refers to a health care professional's failure to exercise due care. Legally, medical negligence (also known as *malpractice*) has four key components: 1) a duty to the patient to provide a certain standard of care; 2) breach in the standard of care; 3) patient injury; and 4) evidence that the breach in the standard of care caused the injury.

Medical Service Organization (MSO)

See: **Management Service Organization (MSO)**

M

Medical Supplies

See also:
Resources

Items which, due to their therapeutic or diagnostic characteristics, are essential in carrying out the care which the physician has ordered for the treatment of a patient's illness or injury. Examples of medical supplies include: catheters, needles, syringes, surgical dressings, irrigating solutions, intravenous fluids, etc.

Medically Indigent

See also:
Underinsurance;
Uninsured

A person whose income and resources are insufficient to pay, either directly or through a health insurance program, the full cost of his/her own health care.

Medically Induced Disease

See: **Iatrogenic Disease**

Medically Necessary

See also:
Appropriate;
Appropriateness Review

Those covered services required to preserve and maintain the health status of a plan member in accordance with the accepted standards of medical practice in the medical community in the area where services are rendered. In other words, services or treatments are considered medically necessary and *appropriate* if they could not have been omitted without adversely affecting the patient's condition or the quality of medical care provided.

Medicare

See also:
Hospital Insurance Program (HI);
Prospective Payment System (PPS);
Supplementary Medical Insurance Program (SMI);
Title XVIII

A federally administered health insurance program for persons aged 65 and older and certain disabled people under 65 years old. Created in 1965 under *Title XVIII* of the Social Security Act, Medicare covers the cost of hospitalization, medical care, and some related services for eligible persons without regard to income. Medicare has two parts: *Medicare Part A: Hospital Insurance (HI) Program* is compulsory and covers inpatient hospitalization costs (currently reimbursed using the *prospective payment system)* and post-hospital care. Medicare also pays for pharmaceuticals provided in hospitals, but not for drugs provided in outpatient settings. *Medicare Part B: Supplementary Medical Insurance Program* is voluntary and covers medically necessary physicians' services, outpatient hospital services (currently reimbursed retrospectively) and a number of other medical services and supplies not covered by Part A. Part B is available for a small premium.

Medicare Cost Report

See also:
Medicare Risk Contract

A report required by HCFA of HMOs that participate in *Medicare Risk contracts.* The Medicare cost report shows the costs for health services provided to Medicare members. Costs are determined on the basis of a ratio of Medicare services to total services applied to total costs.

Medicare Economic Index (MEI)

See also:
Geographic Practice Cost Index (GPCI)

An index used by HCFA to determine limits on physicians' prevailing charges for Medicare reimbursement. The MEI is based on estimates of the expenses of producing physician office services and a measure of increases in earning levels in the economy as a whole.

Medicare / Medicaid Fraud and Abuse Statute

See also:
Safe Harbor Regulations

A federal statute which makes it illegal to knowingly and willfully pay, solicit, or receive any remuneration, directly or indirectly, in return for furnishing or arranging for any health care services for which payment may be made by Medicare or Medicaid. Violation of this provision is a felony, punishable by a fine of up to $25,000, imprisonment for up to five years, or both. Also known as the *anti-kickback statute.*

Medicare Part A

See: **Hospital Insurance Program (HI)** and **Medicare**

Medicare Part B

See: **Supplementary Medical Insurance Program (SMI)** and **Medicare**

M

Medicare Risk Contract

See also:
Adjusted Average Per Capita Cost (AAPCC); Medicare

A type of managed care arrangement whereby the federal government prepays HMOs and competitive medical plans (CMP) for services provided to Medicare beneficiaries who join the managed care plans and agree to receive all their care through the plans. Monthly fixed payments are made by the government to the plans. Payments are based on a percentage of the *adjusted average per capita cost (AAPCC)*. Thus, the HMOs and CMPs are "at risk" (i.e., financially liable) for Medicare services regardless of the extent, expense, or intensity of services rendered.

Medicare SELECT

See also:
Medicare;
Medicare Supplement Policy

A managed care program initiated by the federal government in 1990 for a 3-year period, which permits companies that offer *Medicare supplement policies* (also called *MediGap insurance)* to offer a PPO-type product in conjunction with their MediGap insurance. In exchange for reduced premiums, Medicare beneficiaries receive a financial incentive to use the PPO's network of providers. For example, Medicare SELECT will pay 20% coinsurance if the Medicare beneficiary uses a participating provider. However, the plan pays either no coinsurance or a reduced amount if care is received from a non-participatory provider. Medicare will still pay its share (80%) of the cost of care regardless of whether a network or non-network provider is used.

Medicare Supplement Policy

See also:
Omnibus Budget Reconciliation Act of 1990 (OBRA)

A voluntary, contributory private health insurance policy designed to supplement Medicare benefits, i.e., to "fill the gap" between government reimbursement and provider charges. Most Medicare beneficiaries have some type of private hospital or medical policy to supplement Medicare coverage. The *Omnibus Budget Reconciliation Act of 1990 (OBRA)* standardized Medicare supplement policies into a set of just ten plans that private insurers are allowed to offer. Also called *MediGap Insurance.*

Medicare-Insured Group (MIG)

See also:
Medicare;
Medicare Risk Contract

A type of health care agreement between the federal government and employers or unions, whereby Medicare pays a fixed per capita amount in exchange for the employer or union paying Medicare-covered health services for retirees and Medicare-eligible employees in addition to any supplemental benefits usually provided by the group plan. MIGs are an attempt by the federal government to control costs and integrate Medicare with employment-based group plans. MIGs are similar in some respects to *Medicare Risk* HMOs, except that MIGs operate on a group basis and are not subject to the individual enrollment selection biases of Medicare Risk HMOs.

Medicredit

See: **Tax Credit**

MediGap Insurance

See: **Medicare Supplement Policy**

Member

See also:
Dependent;
Enrollee;
Subscriber

An individual who has enrolled in a health care plan as a subscriber, or a dependent of a subscriber, and for whom the plan has accepted the responsibility for providing health services as specified in the health plan contract. Sometimes called *enrollee* or *subscriber.* A distinction should be noted between the terms *member* and *subscriber*. A subscriber is always a plan member, but a plan member is not necessarily the subscriber, as in the case of a subscriber's dependent.

Member Category

A grouping of health plan members who are broadly classified, usually by age, in order to determine provider reimbursement levels in a capitation environment. At a minimum, the categories are pediatrics, adults, and Medicare. Also called *member type.*

Member Months (MM)

See also:
Per Member Per Month (PMPM)

A count of the total number of months that each plan member is covered. Each member month (MM) is the equivalent of one member for whom the managed care plan is owed (or has been paid) one month's premium income. Member months accumulate for year-to-date statistical purposes.

Members Per Year

See also:
Member Month (MM)

The number of members effective in a health plan on a yearly basis. The calculation is: *member months (MM)* divided by 12.

Mental Health/ Substance Abuse (MH/SA)

See also:
Carve-Out Service; Specialty Network

Refers to psychiatric illnesses and behavioral problems requiring specialized clinical treatments by trained professionals from various disciplines. Managed MH/SA plans may include inpatient, residential, and/ or outpatient services, such as: psychiatric hospitalization and alternatives to psychiatric hospitalization (e.g., residential mental health program, partial confinement treatment program, night care treatment program), restrictive treatment for substance abuse, detoxification and rehabilitation programs, goal-directed psychotherapy, crisis intervention, etc. Traditional indemnity plans and many HMOs usually limit MH/SA coverage to inpatient hospital care and minimal outpatient care, also to certain types of disorders and treatments and to certain types of providers. Some managed care plans offer MH/SA coverage as a *carve-out service* or a *specialty network.*

Metropolitan Statistical Area (MSA)

Refers to a geographical area consisting of a population center and the adjacent communities which have a high degree of economic and social interaction with that center. Specifically, as defined by the U.S. Census Bureau, an MSA must include one city with 50,000 or more inhabitants or an urbanized area with a total population density for the city and surrounding communities of at least 100,000. (For New England MSAs, the population density is 75,000 instead of 100,000.)

Mid-Level Practitioner (MLP)

See also:
Allied Health Professional; Primary Care Physician / Practitioner (PCP)

Refers to professionally trained non-physician providers who deliver medical care, usually under the supervision of a physician but for less cost. MLPs include physician assistants, nurse practitioners, certified nurse midwives, etc. Sometimes called *primary care practitioners (PCP).*

Military Health Services System (MHSS)

See also:
Civilian Health and Medical Program of the Uniformed Services (CHAMPUS)

A large, complex health care system which provides medical services and support directly and indirectly to members of the armed forces, their dependents, and others entitled to Department of Defense medical care. Health care services are provided directly during military operations and ongoing at over 1,000 medical and dental military treatment facilities worldwide. The MHSS also provides care indirectly to beneficiaries through the *CHAMPUS* program.

Minimum Premium Plan (MPP)

See also:
Self-Funded Plan

A financing arrangement for a health benefits program whereby an insurer handles a self-insured employer's claims administration and, for a separate fee, insures against large claims. The employer funds a "bank account," which the insurer draws upon for the payment of claims. The employer is responsible for funding most benefits and the insurer assumes liability for benefits above a predetermined level. Premiums are substantially reduced because the insurer is responsible for funding only a portion of the benefits, which creates a significant cash flow advantage for the employer. Also, since the amounts paid from the fund are not considered insurance, the employer escapes state taxes on premiums.

Miscellaneous Services

See: **Ancillary Services**

M

Mixed Model Managed Care Plan

See also:
Closed Panel;
Hybrid HMO;
Open Panel

A type of managed care plan which uses two or more modes of service delivery. For example, a mixed model HMO may have a *closed panel* system in which enrollees can see only a limited, exclusive panel of providers for routine care, and an *open panel* system which permits members to see private physicians who have contracted individually with the managed care plan. Sometimes called a *hybrid HMO*.

Model HMO Act

See also:
HMO Act;
National Association of Insurance Commissioners (NAIC)

A set of regulatory guidelines for HMOs developed by the *National Association of Insurance Commissioners (NAIC)* in 1972. The Model HMO Act, which now serves as a model for a majority of states' HMO statutes, requires HMOs to effectively provide or arrange for the provision of basic health care services on a prepaid basis and assure that the health care services provided to enrollees are rendered under reasonable standards of care consistent with prevailing professionally recognized standards of medical practice. The NAIC, along with the National Association of HMO Regulators, continues to develop new regulatory guidelines for the HMO industry.

Modified Community Rating

See also:
Community Rating by Class (CRC)

A method of separately rating medical service utilization in a specific geographic area (i.e., in a community) using various demographic characteristics, such as age, sex, marital status, etc., for determining premium rate structures. Sometimes referred to as *community rating by class (CRC).*

Monitoring

See also:
Continuous Quality Improvement (CQI);
Quality Assurance (QA)

An ongoing process for determining that corrective actions instituted to resolve an identified problem in patient services has resulted in sustained resolution of the identified problem. Monitoring is a key component of *quality assurance (QA)* and *continuous quality improvement (CQI)* programs.

Monthly Operating Report (MOR)

A management tool frequently used by well-run managed care organizations to monitor the financial and membership status of their plans. Because managed care is such a dynamic industry, managers need current and reliable operating information. Consequently, MORs are regarded as far more useful than quarterly reports.

Morbidity

See also:
Morbidity Tables; Quality Indicator

The relative incidence (i.e., number of cases) and severity of illness, injury, and disability in a defined population. Morbidity is usually expressed as either general or specific rates of incidence. *Morbidity tables* are developed annually by the U.S. Department of Health and Human Services, based on the average number of illnesses occurring in a large group of persons. Morbidity is considered a *quality indicator* by many health care researchers for measuring quality of care.

Morbidity Table

See also:
Morbidity

A statistical table showing the average number of illnesses, injuries or disabilities affecting a large group of persons. Morbidity tables are prepared annually by the U.S. Health and Human Services Department.

Mortality

See also:
Quality Indicator

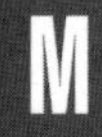

The term means death, literally. Mortality is used to describe the death rate (i.e., probability of death and survival) for a population unit at each age as determined from prior experience. Mortality may be expressed in general terms, such as total number of deaths relative to total population during a year, or as rates specific for diseases or some demographic attribute, such as age, sex, etc. Mortality may be used as a *quality indicator* for measuring the quality of care.

Multidisciplinary

A method for determining treatment plans and delivering care through several practitioners with a wide range of specialties. Often, a multidisciplinary approach is used in complicated cases involving several body systems.

Multiple Employer Trust (MET)

See also:
Multiple Employer Welfare Association (MEWA)

A self-funded legal trust established by a health plan sponsor which brings together employers (usually small employers in the same or related industries) and allows them to provide affordable group health benefits to their respective employees on either an insured or a self-funded basis. METs usually are set up by brokers for the sole purpose of issuing group insurance. Without a MET, many sole proprietorships, partnerships, and small businesses with few employees would be unable to purchase group health insurance.

Multiple Employer Welfare Association (MEWA)

See also:
Multiple Employer Trust (MET)

A group of employers (generally small companies) who form an association for the purpose of purchasing group health insurance. The health plan is usually self-funded, which enables the employers to avoid state mandates and insurance regulation. MEWAs have enabled many small employers to obtain cost-effective health coverage for their employees. However, the self-funded approach can be risky because it requires sufficient financial resources to withstand the risk of high medical costs. MEWAs that fail leave plan members without insurance or recourse.

Multiple Option Plan

See also:
Major Medical Insurance;
Point-of-Service Plan (POS);
Triple Option Plan

A type of group health plan which offers employees several health plan options from which to choose. Typically, the options include an HMO, a PPO, and a *major medical indemnity insurance* plan. Also known as a *triple option plan* or a *point-of-service plan (POS).*

Multispecialty Group (MSG)

See also:
Group Practice

A group of physicians representing two or more medical specialties who work together in a *group practice* setting. Participating physicians typically share equipment, personnel, office expenses, etc., as well as profits.

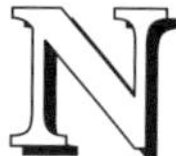

N

National Association for Home Care (NAHC)

See also:
Home Healthcare Agency (HHA);
Hospice Care

A national trade association for providers of home health and hospice care services. Associate memberships are open to businesses, corporations, and others that supply products or services to home care and hospice providers. NAHC offers educational and networking oportunities through an annual meeting, ten regional conferences, and an annual legislative and regulatory conference and computer exposition. Its publications include a weekly and biweekly newsletters, monthly Caring Magazine and Homecare News, and health care reform updates.
Address: NAHC, 519 C Street, NE,
Washington, DC 20002-5809
Phone: (202) 547-7424; Fax: (202) 547-3540

National Association of Employee Benefit Administrators (NAEBA)

See also:
COBRA;
Third Party Administrator (TPA)

A trade association of independent *third party administrator* firms that specialize in design, administration, and reporting of self-funded group health plans, utilization management, and managed care programs. NAEBA offers members advisory assistance in *COBRA* and other regulatory matters, provides educational services, e.g., employee benefits communication program, and access to a nationwide network of PPOs. Member firms subscribe to common standards of practice and utilize a common technology for claims processing.
Address: NAEBA, 12416 S. Harlem Avenue,
Palos Heights, IL 60463
Phone: (708) 448-8077; Fax: (708) 448-8158

National Association of Insurance Commissioners (NAIC)

See also:
Model HMO Act

A trade organization of state insurance regulators which provides a forum for developing national uniformity in the regulation of insurance. NAIC develops model laws, regulations, and guidelines for insurance companies, prepaid managed care plans, and state legislatures. For example, NAIC adopted the *Model HMO Act* in 1972, which authorizes the establishment of HMOs and provides for an ongoing regulatory monitoring system. NAIC also adopted a PPO Arrangements Model Act, which has regulatory requirements applicable to PPO-type products underwritten or administered by insurance companies. NAIC also monitors federal activity which affects insurance regulation, maintains market-based information systems, produces consumer guides, conducts research, provides educational programs, performs solvency surveillance and financial regulation, and offers an accreditation program.
Address: NAIC, 120 W. 12th St., Suite 1100,
Kansas City, MO 64105
Phone: (816) 842-3600; Fax: (816) 471-7004

National Association of Managed Care Physicians (NAMCP)

A professional organization representing physicians who practice in a managed care environment. NAMCP provides a forum for managed care physicians to communicate concerns about the changing health care environment, facilitates physicians' integration into managed care delivery systems, and fosters continuous improvement in the quality of care through research, communication, and education. Members include physicians, medical directors, health care professionals employed by or contracting with managed care plans, and employers interested in managed care.
Address: NAMCP, Innsbrook Corporate Center,
5040 Sadler Rd., Suite 103, Glen Allen, VA 23060-6124
Phone: (804) 527-1905; Fax: (804) 747-5316

National Business Coalition Forum on Health (NBCFH)

See also:
Business Coalition

A national organization representing over 70 non-profit *business coalitions* nationwide with a mission of community-based health care reform. NBCFH supports federal and state reform initiatives, consumer education and responsibility, universal coverage funded through tax credits and tax deductions, and improved measurement systems that enable health care purchasers to compare performance of providers. The organization promotes community-based health reform to employers in cities where business coalitions have not yet emerged, involves providers in the collection and analysis of information on quality, costs, and improvement of the community's health, ensures that health benefit plans contain consumer incentives to use high-value providers, and informs policymakers of the importance of community-based health care reform.
Address: NBCFH, 1015 18th Street, NW, Suite 450, Washington, DC 20036
Phone: (202) 775-9300; Fax: (202) 775-1569

National Center for Policy Analysis (NCPA)

See also:
Tax Credit

A non-profit, non-partisan public policy research institute which supports a "limited government" approach to government regulation and control. NCPA has developed a national health reform plan whereby consumers save for minor medical expenses through individual, portable medical savings accounts (Medisave accounts). Under this plan, consumers can set aside a certain amount of tax-free money each year. Whatever is not used during the year is returned to the consumer. Individuals who purchase health insurance with their own money would receive a *tax credit*, called a *Medicredit*. Employers could continue to offer a wide variety of plans.
Address: NCPA, 12655 N. Central Expressway, Suite 720, Dallas, TX 75243-1739
Phone: (214) 368-6272; Fax: (214) 386-0924

National Committee for Quality Assurance (NCQA)

See also:
Accreditation;
Health Plan Employer Data and Information Set (HEDIS)

An independent, non-profit HMO accrediting organization, composed of independent health care quality experts, employers, labor union officials, and consumer representatives. NCQA's *accreditation* program is designed for most HMO models. Its accreditation standards focus on: 1) quality improvement; 2) credentialing; 3) members' rights and responsibilities; 4) utilization management; 5) preventive health services; 6) medical records. NCQA uses a standardized data reporting system, the *Health Plan Employer Data and Information Set (HEDIS),* to measure HMO quality.
Address: NCQA, 1350 New York Ave., Suite 700, Washington, DC 20005
Phone: (202) 628-5788; Fax: (202) 628-0344

National Drug Code (NDC)

A national classification system for identification of drugs, similar to the Universal Product Code (UPC) used for identification of many commercial products.

National Health Board (NHB)

See also:
American Health Security Act of 1993 (AHSA);
Jackson Hole Group (JHG);
Managed Competition

An independent federal agency proposed as part of several national health care reform plans, including the *American Health Security Act of 1993 (AHSA)* and the *managed competition* model. NHB would oversee development of a national health policy for achieving universal coverage and competition among providers, based on price and quality. The AHSA calls for a seven member board. Members would be nominated by the President with Senate confirmation and serve four-year terms. The NHB would regulate premiums, oversee state health plans, and investigate "unreasonable" increases in drug prices. It would be empowered to expand the standard benefits package, if savings permit. In the managed competition model, three private sector boards sponsored by various user groups would serve as advisors to the NHB.

National Health Expenditures (NHE)

See also:
Gross Domestic Product (GDP)

An economic indicator representing the sum total of expenditures on health care in the United States. The NHE includes: personal health care (hospital and physician, dental, and other professional services, home health care, nursing home care, drugs, medical and non-medical durables, vision products, and other personal health care); administrative costs for health programs, including government public health services; research; and construction. The NHE usually is expressed as a percentage of *gross domestic product (GDP).* For example, the NHE for 1993 was estimated to be $940 billion, or 14% of GDP.

National Health Insurance

A comprehensive system of health care financing which provides uniform health insurance benefits for all or nearly all citizens. National health insurance programs are established by federal law, administered by the federal government, and supported or subsidized by taxation. The term is not yet defined or enacted in the United States, but currently is one of significant political interest. Also called "socialized medicine."

National Health Lawyers Association (NHLA)

A national professional association for attorneys who are interested in or who practice health care law. The NHLA offers members educational, networking, and advocacy opportunities. NHLA also publishes newsletters, texts, references, and other educational materials covering many areas of health law as it relates to managed care. NHLA publications are suitable for the health law "expert" and the "novice."
Address: NHLA, 1620 Eye Street, NW, Suite 900, Washington, DC 20006
Phone: (202) 833-1100; Fax: (202) 833-1105

National HMO

See also:
Blue Cross/Blue Shield Plans (BC/BS);
Health Maintenance Organization (HMO)

A large *health maintenance organization (HMO)* which owns or operates separate HMOs in several states. Examples are Kaiser Permanente, the largest national HMO with 14 HMOs and 6.6 million members, and *Blue Cross/Blue Shield Plans*, with 80 HMOs and 6.2 million members (in 1992).

National Managed Health Care Congress (NMHCC)

A national educational forum which focuses on the entire managed health care industry and its various constituents (e.g., employers, hospitals, physicians, managed care organizations pharmacists, military, MIS vendors). NMHCC seeks to provide common ground in the search for mutually successful solutions among managed care stakeholders. NMHCC holds a national conference in Washington DC in spring and several regional conferences throughout the year.
Address: NMHCC, 1000 Winter Street, Suite 4000, Waltham, MA 02154
Phone: (617) 487-6700; Fax: (617) 487-6709

National Practitioner Data Bank (NPDB)

See also:
Health Care Quality Improvement Act of 1986 (HCQI);
Health Resources and Services Administration (HRSA)

A repository for certain information related to the professional competence and conduct of physicians, dentists, and other health care practitioners. The NPDB was established by the *Health Care Quality Improvement Act of 1986 (HCQI)* to serve as a background reference for health care organizations to check practice records of physicians and practitioners being considered for employment. The HCQI Act requires hospitals, health plans, malpractice insurers, state licensing boards, and professional societies to report malpractice claims settlements, licensure sanctions, and restrictions against practice privileges of a practitioner. NPDB information is confidential, and access is restricted to certain eligible entities. NPDB is administered by the *Health Resources and Services Administration (HRSA),* a federal agency in the Department of Health and Human Services.
Address: NPDB, P.O. Box 6050, Camarillo, CA 93011
Phone: (800) 767-6732

Neonatal Mortality Rate

See also:
Mortality

An index which measures the number of live-born infants who do not reach 28 days of age per 1,000 live births in a given geographical area for a given time period (usually a calendar year).

Neonatal Period

See also:
Neonatal Mortality Rate

The interval from the time of birth up to the time an infant becomes 28 days old. The neonatal period is used for determining *neonatal mortality rates.*

Net Loss Ratio (NLR)

See also:
Loss Ratio

An index which measures an insurance carrier's *loss ratio* after accounting for all expenses. The NLR is calculated as the sum of total claims liability and all expenses divided by premiums.

Network Adequacy

See also:
Managed Care Network;
Network Model HMO;
Provider Panel

Refers to a managed care plan's guidelines for establishing its *provider panel.* Network adequacy guidelines for PPOs and *network model HMOs* may be based on the size, geographical dispersion, and composition (i.e., percentage of primary care physicians) of the *managed care network* of physicians.

Network Model HMO

See also:
Closed Panel;
IPA Model HMO;
Open Panel

A type of HMO which contracts with physician group practices (single or multi-specialty) to form a network (*panel*) of providers to deliver medical services to HMO members. Participating physicians typically work out of their own offices, receive capitated payments for HMO patients, and share in utilization savings. Unlike staff and group model HMOs, network model HMOs may be either *closed panel* or *open panel* plans. In a closed panel plan, the HMO contracts with a limited number of selected group practices. In an open panel plan, participation in the group practices is open to any physician who meets credentialing criteria of the HMO and the physician group. Physicians under contract can also provide services to their non-HMO patients. Similar to an *IPA Model HMO.*

Newborn Boarder Baby

See: **Boarder Baby**

N

Night Care Treatment Program

See also:
Mental Health / Substance Abuse (MH / SA);
Partial Confinement Treatment Program

A type of *partial confinement treatment program* for mental or nervous disorders. Night care treatment programs involve confinement in a hospital or treatment facility during the night, with a room charge. Typically, to qualify as a night care treatment program for reimbursement by plans with such a provision, the program must be available for at least eight hours a night and at least five nights a week.

No Balance Billing Clause

See also:
Hold-Harmless Clause

A term often found in payor-provider contracts (including Medicare contracts with federally qualified HMOs), which states that a provider may not bill a plan member for any balance of the payment owed by the managed care plan regardless of the reason for non-payment. However, the provider may bill the plan member for any amount that the member is required to pay, such as a copayment or coinsurance, or for services not covered under the schedule of benefits. Sometimes called a *hold-harmless clause*.

Non-Cancelable Guaranteed Renewable Policy

See also:
Optionally Renewable Contract

An individual insurance policy under which the covered person has the right to continue his/her coverage until a specified age (e.g., age 65) by the timely payment of premiums. During this period, the insurer cannot unilaterally make any changes in any provision of the policy while it is in force. (Contrast with an *optionally renewable contract*.)

Non-Compliance

See also:
Compliance;
Drug Counseling

The intentional or unintentional misuse (either underutilization or overutilization) of a prescribed drug by an individual who has been placed on drug therapy. Non-compliance often leads to higher health care costs (estimated by the National Pharmaceutical Council to be about $100 billion a year) due to increased hospital admissions, lost productivity on the job, higher outpatient treatment costs, and premature deaths. Underutilization of medications is a serious risk for the elderly and for those on chronic medications that require precise blood levels to be effective, also for individuals with mental or physicial impairments. Non-compliance through drug overutilization, as in the case of patients taking too many sedatives or narcotics, also contributes to higher health care costs due to increased utilization.

Non-Confining Illness

An illness that prevents an insured person from working but does not confine the individual to a hospital or other treatment facility, or to his/her home.

N

Non-Contributory Plan

See also:
Contributory Plan;
Medical Expense Reimbursement Plan (MERP)

Refers to a situation in which the group health plan sponsor (e.g., employer) pays the entire cost of premiums for health plan coverage. Under this type of plan, employees do not contribute any money toward the cost of the coverage. In a non-contributory plan, 100 percent of the eligible employees must be covered. Sometimes called *medical expense reimbursement plan (MERP)*. (Contrast with *contributory plan*.)

Non-Core Coverage

See also:
Core Coverage

Generally, refers to dental and vision benefits, in contrast to *core coverage*, which typically means medical benefits only.

Non-Disabling Injury

An injury that may require medical care but does not result in loss of working time or income.

Non-Occupational Policy

A type of insurance policy that provides coverage for sickness or off-the-job injury. Non-occupational insurance, however, does not cover disability resulting from injury or sickness covered by a Workers' Compensation program. Group accident and sickness policies often are non-occupational insurance policies.

Non-Participatory Provider Indemnity Benefits

See also:
Non-Participatory Provider (NonPar); Point-of-Service Plan (POS)

A type of health care coverage for services rendered by providers who are not under contract with the health plan. Non-participatory provider indemnity benefits typically are offered by *point-of-service (POS)* plans. The benefits are covered on an indemnity (i.e., fee-for-service) basis, and usually carry high copayment requirements and deductibles as a disincentive to using *non-participatory providers.*

Non-Participatory Provider (NonPar)

See also:
Participating Provider

Refers to a provider that has not contracted with an insurance carrier or managed care plan to provide health care services to plan members. A nonpar elects not to be in a plan's managed care network or provider panel. (Contrast with *participating provider.*)

Non-Profit Insurer

An insurance carrier organized under state laws to provide hospital, medical, or dental insurance on a not-for-profit basis. Non-profit insurers are exempt from certain state taxes, like corporate and sales taxes.

Norms

See also:
Standards

Numerical or statistical measures of usual observed performance regarding health care provided to a given number of patients over time. Norms may be used as *standards*. Norms and standards both imply a single value rather than a range of values. For example, a norm can be the mean, the median, or some other cut-off point in a series of values.

Not-for-Profit Facility

See also:
Community Benefits; Voluntary Hospital

Any provider facility (e.g., *voluntary hospital*) which is owned and operated by one or more non-profit corporations or associations, whereby no part of the earnings may benefit any private shareholder or individual. Not-for-profit facilities are exempt from corporate taxes and, in some states, also are exempted from state taxes if they show that a certain percentage of profit is allocated to *community benefits.*

Nurse Practitioner (NP)

See also:
Allied Health Professional; Primary Care Physician / Practitioner (PCP)

A licensed nurse who has completed a nurse practitioner program at the master's or certificate level and is trained in providing primary care services. Generally, nurse practitioners (NP) provide services at a lower cost than *primary care physicians (PCP).* NPs are qualified to carry out expanded health care evaluations and decision-making regarding patient care, including diagnosis, treatment, and prescriptions, usually but not necessarily under a physician's supervision. NPs may be trained in medical specialties, such as pediatrics, geriatrics, and midwifery. Legal barriers in some states prevent NPs from qualifying for direct Medicare and Medicaid reimbursement, writing prescriptions, and admitting patients to hospitals. Also called *advance practice nurse (APN).*

Nursing Care Institution (NCI)

See: **Nursing Home**

Nursing Home
See also:
Intermediate Care Facility (ICF); Skilled Nursing Facility (SNF)

A facility which provides long-term maintenance and personal care to patients with chronic or disabling conditions. Most nursing home patients are elderly and have limited potential for rehabilitation. *Nursing homes* include free-standing institutions and identifiable components of facilities that providie nursing care and related services, such as *skilled nursing, intermediate care,* and long-term care facilities, but not residential care facilities (RCF). Also called *nursing care institution (NCI).*

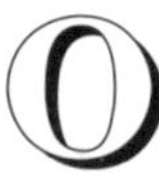

Occupancy Rate
See also:
Bed Day; Patient Day

A measure of inpatient use of a provider facility expressed as the average percentage of days per year that hospital beds are occupied by patients. Occupancy rate is calculated by dividing available *bed days* by *patient days.*

Occupational Disease
See also:
Workers' Compensation (WC)

A disease or health condition resulting from performance of an occupation. In most states, occupational disease is now covered under *workers' compensation (WC)* benefits plans.

Occupational Hazards

See also:
Ergonomic Hazard;
Occupational Disease;
Occupational Safety and Health Act (OSHA)

Risks related to occupations that expose the covered person to greater than normal physical danger by the very nature of the work in which the insured is engaged. Also refers to the varying periods of absence from work that can be expected due to disability resulting from an *occupational disease.*

Occupational Health Services

See also:
Occupational Disease;
Occupational Safety and Health Act (OSHA)

Health services designed to protect the physical, mental, and social well-being of individuals in relation to their jobs and working environments.

Occupational Safety and Health Act (OSHA)

See also:
Occupational Disease;
Occupational Hazard

A federal statute which establishes national standards for health and safety conditions in the workplace. OSHA also provides for the reporting and compiling of statistics pertaining to *occupational diseases* and injuries. The federal agency charged with responsibility for enforcing OSHA is the Occupational Safety and Health Administration (also referred to as *OSHA*), which is part of the Labor Department.

Occupational Therapist (OT)

See also:
Activities of Daily Living (ADL)
Occupational Health Services;
Occupational Therapy

A specially trained health professional who evaluates the self-care and work performance skills of well and disabled individuals. OTs plan and implement programs designed to restore, develop, and maintain patients' abilities to satisfactorily accomplish *activities of daily living (ADL)* required for specific ages and necessary for certain occupational roles. Formal educational preparation requires at least four years of college leading to a baccalaureate degree, plus a minimum of six months' field work.

Occupational Therapy

See also:
Occupational Health Services;
Occupational Therapist (OT)

Medically directed treatment of physically or mentally disabled individuals by means of constructive activities designed by a qualified *occupational therapist (OT)* to promote the restoration of useful function.

Office of Health Maintenance Organizations (OHMO)

See also:
Office of Prepaid Health Care Operations and Oversight (OPHCOO)

The former name for the federal agency within the U.S. Department of Health and Human Services which oversees federal activity relating to HMOs. OHMO has been reorganized, initially as the *Office of Prepaid Health Care (OPHC),* and now as the *Office of Prepaid Health Care Operations and Oversight (OPHCOO).*

O

Office of Personnel Management (OPM)

See also:
Federal Employees Health Benefit Program (FEHBP);
Similarly-Sized Subscriber Group (SSSG)

The federal agency authorized to offer certain choices of health benefits plans to federal employees. (See *Federal Employees Health Benefit Program*) OPM can offer both experience-rated plans and comprehensive community-rated plans (mostly HMOs). OPM does not engage in a competitive bidding process. Instead, it relies on rates set by other managed care contractors and compares OPM rates with other HMO groups of similar size and benefits. HMOs participating in FEHBP are subject to periodic audit by the OPM, which involves reviews of state and federal rate filings, actual billings to commercial accounts, and rate worksheets used in developing the HMO's premium.

Office of Prepaid Health Care Operations and Oversight (OPHCOO)

See also:
Office of Health Maintenance Organizations (OHMO)

A division of the HCFA which is responsible for overseeing federal HMO qualification, CMP eligibility, ongoing HMO and CMP regulation, and employer compliance efforts. OPHCOO also administers Medicare Risk contracts, determines the capitation formula and reimbursement policies, and oversees the operation of the prepaid health information system. HMO qualification and CMP eligibility review processes are complex and can take six months to a year, or longer. Review areas include: legal, financial viability, health services delivery, and marketing. The OPHCOO was once a part of the U.S. Public Health Service, and called the *Office of Health Maintenance Organizations (OHMO).*
Address: OPHCOO, Cohen Building, Room 4406,
330 Independence Ave., SW, Washington, DC 20201
Phone: (202) 619-0845; Fax: (202) 619-2011

Office Visit

See also:
Encounter

An *encounter* between a plan member and a health care professional which requires the patient to travel from his/her home to the professional's usual place of practice. Also may refer to the professional services provided in an outpatient setting.

Omnibus Reconciliation Act (OBRA)

See also:
Peer Review Organizations (PRO); Quality Review Committees (QRC); Sixth Omnibus Reconciliation Act of 1985 (SOBRA)

Refers to the *Sixth Omnibus Reconciliation Act of 1985 (SOBRA)*, which created *Quality Review Committees (QRC)* and empowered QROs and *Peer Review Organizations (PRO)* to monitor quality of care for Medicare recipients enrolled in HMOs or CMPs. OBRA provided for civil financial penalties for health plans that failed to provide proper care. It also restricted the types of physician incentives that a managed care plan may use when providing care for Medicare beneficiaries. Additionally, OBRA made disenrollment from HMOs and CMPs far easier for Medicare beneficiaries.

On-Site Concurrent Review (OSCR)

See: **Concurrent Review**

Oncology

See also:
Chemotherapy

A branch of medicine that specializes in cancer diagnosis and treatment.

Open Enrollment

See also:
Community Rating;
Evidence of Insurability (E of I);
Waiting Period

An enrollment period (usually annual) during which employees may change their health plans among those offered by their employers without restriction, that is, without *evidence of insurability (E of I)* or a *waiting period*. Typically, the open enrollment period occurs for one month once a year. In some states, open enrollment is a requirement of public programs. In these situations, an HMO must accept any individual, including persons from outside an employer group, regardless of health status. Also, the HMO is required to charge these individuals the standard community rate. This type of open enrollment is referred to as *community open enrollment*. Sometimes called "open season."

O

Open Panel

See also:
IPA Model HMO;
Self-Referral

A type of managed care plan, such as an *IPA model HMO,* which contracts with physicians who operate out of their own offices and allows plan members to see a participating provider without a referral from another physician. In other words, a plan member may *self-refer* to other participating providers.

Open-Ended HMO

See: **Point-of-Service Plan (POS)**

Optimal Achievable

See also:
Practice Guidelines; Quality Improvement Program (QIP)

Refers to the highest level of quality attainable under specified conditions. The term is often used in the development of *practice guidelines* and in *quality improvement programs (QIP)*. Optimal achievable standards often exceed current practices and expectations. However, eventual compliance is viewed as feasible and important in the provision of patient care.

Optionally Renewable Contract

See also:
Non-Cancelable Guaranteed Renewable Policy

A type of health insurance contract in which the insurer reserves the right to terminate coverage at any anniversary date or, in some cases, at any premium due date, but does not have the right to terminate coverage between such dates. (Compare with *non-cancelable guaranteed renewable policy*).

Organized System of Care (OSC)

See: **Integrated Delivery System (IDS)**

O

Osteopathic

See also:
Family Practice; Osteopathic Physician (D.O.)

A branch of medicine that emphasizes normal body mechanics and manipulation techniques for diagnosing and correcting disease and faulty body structure. Osteopathy is based on the theory that the body is capable of making its own remedies against disease and other toxic conditions when it is in normal structural alignment and has favorable environmental conditions and adequate nutrition. *Osteopathic physicians (D.O.)* are graduates of accredited schools of osteopathic medicine and generally practice family medicine.

Other Party Liability (OPL)

See: **Coordination of Benefits (COB)**

Out-of-Area Benefits

See also:
Out-of-Area Services (OOA)

Benefits that an HMO provides to its members when they are outside the HMO's service area. Out-of-area coverage is usually limited to emergency services. Most managed care plans stipulate that out-of-area emergency care services will be provided (and covered) until the plan member can be returned to the plan's service area for medical management of the case.

Out-of-Area Services (OOA)

See also:
Authorization; Non-Participatory Provider (NonPar); Out-of-Area Benefits

Medical services provided to HMO members by non-network (i.e., *non-participatory)* providers when plan members are outside the HMO's service area. Generally, out-of-area services (OOA) are not covered unless a delay in treatment would adversely affect the patient's medical condition. Plan approval (see *authorization*) also must be obtained in order for the out-of-area services to be covered.

Out-of-Network Services (OON)

See also:
After-Hours Care; Non-Participatory Provider (NonPar)

Health care services received by a managed care plan member from a *non-participatory provider (nonpar).* Reimbursement is usually lower when a member goes "out-of-network." Other financial penalties also may apply for out-of-network services.

Out-of-Pocket Limit

See also:
Out-of-Pocket Payments (OOP); Preadmission Certification

The total amount of money that a plan member must pay out of his/her own pocket toward eligible expenses for himself/herself and/or dependents. *Out-of-pocket payments (OOP)* include deductibles, copayments, and coinsurance, as defined in the contract. Once the out-of-pocket limit is reached, benefits increase to 100% for health services received during the rest of that calendar year. Some out-of-pocket costs, such as penalties for not obtaining *preadmission certification*, are not eligible for out-of-pocket limits.

Out-of-Pocket Payments (OOP)

See also:
Cost-Sharing Techniques; Out-of-Pocket Limit

Cash payments made by a plan member or insured person to the provider in the form of deductibles, coinsurance, or copayments during a defined period (usually a calendar year) before plan or the insurer covers all remaining services at 100%.

Outcome Audit

See also:
Outcomes; Process Audit

A type of medical care evaluation that focuses on results of treatment using criteria designed to assess desired patient *outcomes*. (Contrast with *process audit,* which focuses on the components of appropriate clinical intervention rather than desired outcomes.)

Outcomes

See also:
Outcomes Measurement; Outcomes Research; Severity-Adjusted Clinical Outcomes

The end results of medical care, as indicated by recovery, disability, functional status, mortality, morbidity, or patient satisfaction. Outcomes are studied as a means of determining the quality of care rendered by providers. The standard of judgment is the attainment of a specified end result, or "outcome." Disease has a "natural history" that medical care seeks to alter. Thus, desired outcomes would be improved health, lowered mortality and morbidity, alleviation or improvement of abnormal conditions, etc.

Outcomes Management Standards Board (OMSB)

See also:
Managed Competition; National Health Board (NHB)

One of three private sector organizations which would be created in the *managed competition* model for health care reform. OMSB would be responsible for designing and overseeing a national quality reporting system based primarily on patient outcomes measures. The national data base would be used to evaluate quality and performance of providers and insurers, and would also support the continuous updating of effectiveness standards. The other two private sector groups in this model are a Health Standards Board (HSB) and a Health Insurance Standards Board (HISB). These three private sector groups would advise the *National Health Board*, an independent federal agency, regarding national policy.

Outcomes Management System (OMS)

See also:
Health Outcomes Institute; InterStudy; Outcomes Measurement

A standardized method for measuring patient outcomes, which was developed by *InterStudy*, a health research organization. The OMS now is administered by a new health policy research organization, called the *Health Outcomes Institute.* The OMS is a collection of several measures of patient function, well-being and clinical status. The OMS relies on quality-of-life self-assessments by patients who complete a questionnaire and on condition-specific forms filled out by the treating physicians.

Outcomes Measurement

See also:
Outcomes; Quality Indicator; Severity-Adjusted Clinical Outcomes

The process of systematically tracking a patient's clinical treatment and responses to that treatment using generally accepted outcomes measures, or *quality indicators*, such as mortality, morbidity, disability, functional status, recovery, and patient satisfaction. Such measures are considered by many health care researchers as the only valid way to determine the effectiveness of medical care. Some health care professionals say they are the only way to measure the quality of care, too. Outcomes measurement also is used for performing cost-benefit analyses of medical care.

Outcomes Research

See also:
Outcomes Measurement;
Severity-Adjusted Clinical Outcomes

A specialized branch of research which is attempting to identify and develop standards for *severity-adjusted clinical outcomes* of medical services for large groups of patients.

Outflow

See also:
Inflow;
Service Area;
Utilization

The number or proportion of people in a local market or *service area* who leave the area for some health care service. Outflow is a useful measure for forecasting *utilization* of services in a market area because it represents use of out-of-area providers by local residents only. Outflow is usually estimated from a sample survey of local residents. By contrast, *inflow* represents the proportion of total utilization by both residents and non-residents of all local providers in a given area. Like outflow, inflow is also used for forecasting service utilization in a particular area.

Outliers

See also:
Diagnosis-Related Group (DRG);
Trim Points

In *DRGs*, refers to patient cases that fall at either extreme of the bell-shaped normal distribution curve. For example, very short or very long hospital stays, or extraordinarily high or low costs compared with most cases classified in the same DRG, are considered outliers. In such cases, hospitals usually are reimbursed by Medicare (also by some managed care plans) on a per diem basis or for itemized charges instead of the normal DRG rate.

Outpatient Care

See also:
Ambulatory Care;
Outpatient (OP)

Medical services and other related services provided by a hospital or other qualified *ambulatory care* facility or supplier, such as a mental health clinic, rural health clinic, mobile X-Ray unit, free-standing dialysis unit, which does not require admission to the facility for an overnight stay. Examples of outpatient services are physical therapy, diagnostic radiology, laboratory tests, radiation therapy, minor surgeries, etc.

Outpatient (OP)

See also:
Ambulatory Care; Inpatient (IP)

A patient who receives medical services at a health care facility without being admitted to the facility for an overnight stay, that is, on an outpatient basis. The antonym is *inpatient (IP)*.

Outpatient Surgery

See: **Day Surgery** and **Free-Standing Outpatient Surgery Center**

Outreach

See also:
Access

A process of systematically "reaching out" within a community to identify people in need of health care services, alert community members to the availability of services, or facilitate people's entry (i.e., *access*) into the health care service delivery system.

Outside Referral

See also:
Referral

Referral of a plan member to a consultant provider who is not in the plan's network or not within the physician group that is under contract to deliver the managed care plan's professional medical services.

Over-the-Counter Drug (OTC)

See also:
Legend Drug

A drug that is advertised and sold directly to the public without a prescription. An example of an OTC drug is aspirin. The antonym is *prescription drug,* or *legend drug*.

Overhead Insurance

See also:
Short-Term Disability Income Insurance

A type of *short-term disability income insurance* policy, which reimburses the insured for specified, fixed monthly expenses that are normal and customary in the operation and conduct of his/her business.

Overinsurance

See also:
Coordination of Benefits (COB);
Duplication of Benefits;
Underinsurance

Refers to the situation in which a person is covered under more than one plan and thus is eligible for total benefits that exceed actual medical costs. The antonym is *underinsurance*.

Overtreatment

See also:
Appropriate;
Medically Necessary;
Undertreatment

Refers to the provision of more health care services than are consistent with or justified by the diagnosis and treatment plan, being neither *medically necessary* nor *appropriate*. The antonym is *undertreatment*.

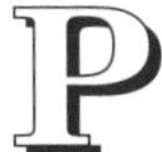

Paid Claims

See also:
Claim

The dollar amounts paid to providers by insurance carriers or plan sponsors for covered hospital, medical, or surgical services. These amounts do not include any member liability for ineligible charges, deductibles, or copayments.

Paid Claims Loss Ratio (PCLR)

See also:
Loss Ratio;
Paid Claims;
Premium

A financial measure used by managed care plans and insurers to compare actual paid claims to the premiums paid. The PCLR is calculated by dividing *paid claims* by *premiums*.

Partial Confinement Treatment Program

See also:
Mental Health / Substance Abuse (MH / SA);
Night Care Treatment Program

A planned mental health or substance abuse treatment program operated by a hospital or psychiatric treatment facility in which clinical services are provided on less than a full-time inpatient basis. Generally, partial confinement treatment programs are supervised by a psychiatric physician who reviews the program and periodically (typically, at least once a week) evaluates its effectiveness. Often, this type of partial confinement program is implemented as an alternative or follow-up to inpatient hospital care. A *night care treatment program* is an example of a partial confinement treatment program.

Partial Disability

See also:
Residual Disability Benefit;
Total Disability

A physicial condition resulting from an injury or illness which prevents a covered person from performing one or more of the functions of his/her regular job.

Partial Hospitalization

See also:
Partial Confinement Treatment Program;
Night Care Treatment Program

A formal therapeutic program which provides less than 24 hour care (usually during the day, but also may be during the night) in a hospital or other type of provider institution, such as a mental health facility, rehabilitation hospital, or intermediate care facility for patients in transition from full-time inpatient care to outpatient care and a return to an active daily life in the community.

Participating Provider

See also:
Preferred Provider;
Provider Panel

A provider who has contracted with a managed care plan to provide medical services to plan members. The provider may be a hospital or other medical facility, a pharmacy, a physician, or other practitioner who has contractually accepted the terms and conditions as set forth by the plan. Also called a *preferred provider.*

Participation

Refers to the number of eligible employees or group members enrolled in a health plan. Participation is usually identified as a percentage relative to the total eligible population. For example, a 75% participation requirement for a group health plan means that at least 75% of eligible employees and eligible dependents must enroll for coverage in the plan.

Patient Days

See also:
Average Daily Census (ADC);
Average Length of Stay (ALOS);
Occupancy Rate

Refers to each calendar day of care provided to a hospital inpatient under the terms of the patient's health plan, but excluding the day of discharge. "Patient days" is a measure of institutional use and usually is stated as the accumulated total number of inpatients (excluding newborns) each day for a given reporting period, tallied at a specified time (like midnight) per 1000 use rate, or patient days/1000. A day of routine nursery care provided to a newborn during the mother's stay usually is not counted as a patient day because newborn care is considered part of the obstetrical care provided to the mother. Patient days are calculated by multiplying admissions by *average length of stay (ALOS).*

Patient Origin Study

See also:
Catchment Area;
Market Area

A type of study for determining the geographical distribution of the homes of patients served by a particular provider facility, managed care plan, or health program. Generally, patient origin studies are conducted by providers, managed care organizations, and health planning agencies to help define their respective *catchment areas* or *market areas.*

Payer (Payor)

See also:
Managed Care Network (MCN);
Third Party Payor

Refers to any managed care organization, third party administrator, employer, association, trust fund, insurance carrier, the federal government, or other entity that is liable for health care coverage for plan members. Payers often enter into agreements with *managed care networks* to provide certain financial incentives encouraging plan members to use participating providers. The term may be spelled both ways, as *payer* and as *payor*.

Payor Profile

See also:
Payer (Payor);
Third Party Payor

An analysis of a *third party payor*, such as a managed care plan, third party administrator, or insurance company for evaluation, comparison or contract management purposes. Typically, a payor profile includes information about the types of plans, products, and services offered by the company, its financial performance, network development philosophy, participating providers and their locations, steerage incentives, preferred reimbursement arrangements, rate structures, data analysis capabilities, etc.

Peer Review

See also:
Peer Review Organization (PRO)

An evaluation by practicing physicians or other clinical professionals of the appropriateness, effectiveness, and efficiency of medical services ordered or performed by other practicing physicians or professionals. Usually, the term refers to the quality assurance activities of *Peer Review Organizations (PRO),* which review services provided to Medicare and Medicaid beneficiaries and sometimes to members of managed care plans. A peer review focuses on how well services are performed by all health personnel involved in the delivery of the care under review, and how appropriate the services are to meet the patients needs.

Peer Review Organization (PRO)

See also:
Peer Review;
Professional Standards Review Organization (PRSO);
Tax Equity and Fiscal Responsibility Act of 1982 (TEFRA)

A federal program established by the *Tax Equity and Fiscal Responsibility Act of 1982 (TEFRA),* which monitors the medical necessity and quality of services provided to Medicare and Medicaid beneficiaries under the prospective payment reimbursement system. PROs also validate provider coding assignments that affect Medicare reimbursement. In 1984, HCFA began contracting with peer review organizations (PRO) in every state. Hospitals are required to contract with a PRO in its state as a condition of receiving Medicare payments. PRO reviews evaluate care provided by hospitals, hospital outpatient departments, ambulatory surgical centers, emergency rooms, skilled nursing facilities, home health agencies, risk-sharing HMOs and competitive medical plans. Along with utilization and quality reviews, PROs are also responsible for investigating complaints by Medicare beneficiaries regarding the quality of care provided by HMOs. PROs are held responsible for maintaining and lowering admission rates, reducing lengths of stay, and ensuring against inadequate treatment.

Pended for Review

See also:
Authorization

In claims processing, refers to a case which does not have the issue of *authorization* resolved. When a case is pended for review, the processing of the claim is temporarily suspended until the case undergoes a medical or administrative review, which usually results in retrospective authorization.

Per Contract Per Month (PCPM)

See: **Per Member Per Month (PMPM)**

Per Diem Reimbursement

See also:
Adverse Selection

A managed care reimbursement arrangement based on a set rate per day per plan member rather than on charges for services provided, as in *fee-for-service reimbursement.* In a "global per diem" arrangement, the hospital aggregates individual services into a uniform daily rate based on average costs for all admissions, and then bills the managed care plan an all-inclusive rate per day of care. *Adverse selection* can be a risk under this arrangement because the global per diem is based on an assumption that the plan's enrollees will require a certain blend of medical-surgical and intensive care unit (ICU) days. If, for example, there is heavier than expected ICU usage, the hospital loses money. In a "multiple per diem" arrangement, the hospital negotiates separate daily rates for different medical services, e.g., med-surg, ICU, oncology, etc.

Per Member Per Month (PMPM)

See also:
Member Months (MM)

A unit of measure used by prepaid health plans (typically HMOs) to describe capitation payments. PMPM may relate to either revenues or costs expressed in terms of each effective member of a plan for each month that the member was effective. It is calculated by dividing the number of plan members (in terms of of revenues) by *member months (MM).* Sometimes called *per contract per month (PCPM).*

Per Thousand Members Per Year (PTMPY)

See also:
Utilization

A method commonly used by managed care plans for reporting *utilization* of health services by plan members. For example, hospital utilization is usually expressed as days *per thousand members per year.*

Percentile

See also:
Maximum Allowable Payment (MAP)

A distribution range of provider charges, as determined by a third party payor for specific services. Managed care plans frequently use the percentile method for determining the *maximum allowable payment (MAP)* for various covered services. For example, if a plan uses the 90th percentile for setting its MAP, payment is made for any charge at or below the 90th percentile level of charges.

Performance Standards

See also:
Productivity; Standards

Refers to measures which have been set by competent authority and used by managed care plans as rules for determining the level of quality that a provider is expected to meet. Performance standards may define level of medical care or volume of care delivered per time period. For example, performance standards for an obstetrician/gynecologist may specify: office hours, office visits per week, on-call day, deliveries per year, gynecological operations per year, etc.

Pharmaceutical Manufacturers Association (PMA)

A national trade association representing the interests of more than 100 research-based pharmaceutical companies. PMA supports public policies that foster private research and development, free trade principles, and full protection of intellectual property rights. PMA studies the medical, social, and economic benefits provided by specific drugs and by the pharmaceutical industry in general, and communicates this information to policy-makers and the public. PMA favors a managed competition approach to health care reform, inclusion of prescription drug benefits in the standard benefit package, and voluntary efforts by drug companies rather than government price controls and global budgets to restrain price increases.
Address: PMA, 100 15th Street, NW,
Washington, DC 20005
Phone: (202) 835-3400; Fax: (202) 785-4834

Pharmacy and Therapeutics Committee (P&T)

See also:
Drug Formulary

An organized panel of pharmacists and physicians from varyious practice specialties, who serve as an advisory panel to a managed care plan regarding safe and effective use of prescription medications. A major function of the P&T committee is to develop, manage and administer *drug formularies.*

Pharmacy Services Administration Organization (PSAO)

See also:
Preferred Providers

A network of pharmacists that contracts with employers, insurance carriers, or third party administrators to provide drug dispensing and pharmacy services for members of a managed care plan. Plan members are encouraged through cost incentives to use these *preferred providers* for pharmacy services.

Physician

See also:
Doctor of Osteopathy (D.O.);
Primary Care Physician (PCP)

A health care professional who is qualified by education, authorized by law, and duly licensed to practice medicine, that is, provide the full spectrum of diagnostic and therapeutic services to patients. In the United States, physicians may be either medical doctors (M.D.) or *doctors of osteopathy (D.O.).*

Physician Contingency Reserve (PCR)

See also:
Participating Physician; Withhold

The "at-risk" portion of a claim which is deducted and withheld by the managed care plan before payment is made to a *participating physician* for medical services provided to a plan member. The PCR is intended to serve as an incentive for appropriate utilization and quality of care. The amount (usually 20% of the claim) remains within the plan and is credited to the doctor's account. Money in the PCR can be used when the plan needs funds to pay for claims. The withheld money may be returned to the physician in varying amounts, which are determined based on analysis of his/her performance or productivity compared against his/her peers. Also called a *withhold.*

Physician Extender

See: **Physician's Assistant (PA)**

Physician's Assistant (PA)

See also:
Allied Health Professional

A specially trained and licensed (where necessary), or otherwise credentialed *allied health professional*, who performs certain medical procedures previously reserved to the physician. PAs usually practice under the supervision of a physician. Sometimes called a *physician extender.*

Physician's Current Procedural Terminology, 4th Edition (CPT-4)

See also:
Current Procedural Terminology (CPT); HCFA Common Procedure Coding System (HCPCS)

A classification system which assigns a unique five-digit code to medical procedures and services performed by physicians and other practitioners. CPT-4 codes usually are used by physicians for procedure identification and billing purposes. The CPT-4 coding system has become the health care industry's standard for the reporting of medical procedures and services. An important advantage of the CPT-4 system is that it permits effective communication and comparison of physician services nationwide.

Physician-Hospital-Community Organization (PHCO)

See also:
Physician-Hospital Organization (PHO)

A legal entity formed by one or more local hospitals, a group of physicians, and community organizations to further mutual interests and achieve market objectives. Community representatives sit on the board, along with physicians and hospital representatives. PHCOs function similarly as Physician-Hospital Organizations (PHO) and, like PHOs, usually are organized for the purpose of obtaining managed care contracts directly with employers. The PHCO serves as a collective negotiating and contracting unit.

Physician-Hospital Organization (PHO)

See also:
Hospital-Physician Arrangement (HPA); Physician-Hospital-Community Organization (PHCO)

A legal entity formed by a hospital and a group of physicians to further mutual interests and achieve market objectives. PHOs are usually organized for the purpose of obtaining managed care contracts directly with employers. The PHO serves as a collective negotiating and contracting unit. Generally, physicians in a PHO maintain ownership of their practices and agree to accept managed care patients according to the terms of a professional services agreement with the PHO. PHOs are one of the few managed care arrangements that offer physicians opportunities for substantial participation in management, governance, and operations. For hospitals, PHOs offer opportunities to form a more unified medical staff, more effectively market medical services to payors, and enhance physician relationships overall. In some cases, the community is included as a part of the legal entity. Then the organization is called a *physician-hospital-community organization (PHCO).* In this type of organization, community representatives also sit on the board, along with physicians and hospital representatives.

Place of Service

The site where health services are provided, such as a physician's office, hospital, clinic, home, etc.

Plan Sponsor

The group that organizes a health plan, and/or finances its facilities, and/or makes up its governing board. For example, an employer that offers its employees health benefits through a group health plan is the plan sponsor.

Point-of-Service Plan (POS)

See also:
Dual Option; Multiple Option Plan

A type of managed care plan in which members are given a choice as to how to receive services, whether through an HMO, PPO, or fee-for-service plan, at the time when the medical services are needed (i.e., at the "point of service"). For example, under a *dual option* plan, which enrolls its members in both an HMO and an indemnity plan, members receive benefits at a greater level if they use participating providers than if they choose an out-of-network, or non-participatory, provider (e.g., 100% vs. 70% coverage). Also called *open-ended HMO, swing-out HMO*, *self-referral option*, or *multiple option plan.*

Policyholder

See also:
Master Group Contract

Under a group health plan, the policyholder may be the employer, labor union, or trustee to whom the *master group contract* is issued. In a plan that contracts directly with an individual or family, the policyholder is the individual to whom the contract is issued.

Pooling

See also:
Risk Pool

The process of combining all claims or cost experience for defined populations (e.g., all groups with more than ten but fewer than fifty insured persons) or types of coverage (e.g., school, business) into one *risk pool* in order to spread the risk, or claims liability.

Positron Emission Tomography (PET)

See also:
Ancillary Services

A relatively new "high tech" diagnostic procedure used primarily for detecting blockage in the coronary arteries. PET is considered a high-cost, non-invasive, experimental *ancillary service* by many managed care plans. A single test costs approximately $2,500 and, currently, is not reimbursed by Medicare, CHAMPUS, or most health plans.

Practice Guidelines

See also:
Optimal Achievable; Practice Pattern; Provider Profiling; Standards

These are recommended, codified procedures and techniques for the treatment of specific illnesses and medical conditions in order to obtain *optimal achievable* results. Practice guidelines are being developed by medical societies and medical research organizations, such as the American Medical Association (AMA) and the Agency for Health Care Policy and Research (AHCPR), as well as many HMOs, insurers, and business coalitions. Practice guidelines are not rigid *standards* that must be followed. Rather, they are designed to serve as educational support for physicians, and also as quality assurance and accountability measures for managed care plans.

Practice Pattern

See also:
Practice Guidelines; Provider Profiling

Refers to the usual manner or pattern by which an individual physician uses medical resources to treat patients. Physicians with similar training, who treat similar patients in comparable practice settings, may vary considerably in the extent that they prescribe medications, order laboratory, X-ray, or other diagnostic tests, hospitalize patients, use consulting specialists, delegate to non-physician personnel, etc. Thus, each physician develops his/her own unique practice pattern. More and more, hospitals, managed care plans, and some health care purchasers are evaluating and monitoring physician practice patterns in an attempt to identify and control the heavy resource users in order to contain costs.

Practitioner

See also:
Clinician

A health care professional who is qualified in the clinical practice of medicine, psychiatry, psychology, or other allied health profession, as distinguished from one specializing in laboratory or research techniques. Also called *clinician.*

Pre-established Criteria

See also:
Performance Standards;
Standards;
Utilization Review (UR)

Written criteria or guidelines that are accepted *standards* of health care or practice. Utilization review organizations (URO) use pre-established criteria in their evaluations of appropriateness, quality, and medical necessity of services provided to members of managed care plans.

Pre-existing Condition

See also:
American Health Security Act of 1993;
Exclusions

Any physical or mental health condition, including injury or disease, that occurred and has been diagnosed or treated within a specified period of time prior to enrollment in a health plan. Many insurance carriers and managed care plans refuse to cover members' claims related to pre-existing conditions. Federally qualified HMOs, however, cannot limit coverage for pre-existing conditions for groups, but can limit coverage for individual policies. In President Clinton's proposal for health care reform, called the *American Health Security Act of 1993*, all health plans would be unable to refuse or limit coverage for pre-existing conditions.

Preadmission Certification

See also:
Authorization;
Prospective Review;
Utilization Management (UM)

A *utilization management (UM)* technique used by managed care organizations to ensure that only those plan members who need hospital care are admitted to the hospital. Preadmission certification is usually done before admission for non-emergency care, or shortly after admission for emergency care. As part of the preadmission certification process, an estimated length of stay (LOS) is established in conjunction with the admission process, and is then used to monitor the patient's LOS during the course of his/her hospitalization.

Preadmission Review See: **Prospective Review**

Preadmission Screening Program (PAS)

See also:
Long-Term Care (LTC)

A managed care technique used by state-administered Medicaid programs to manage *long-term care* costs and utilization for nursing homes. Medicaid PAS programs vary from state to state. However, they usually include a comprehensive on-site assessment of the patient's needs, including an evaluation of physical and mental health, functional status, and social supports. A recommendation also is made concerning what long-term care services are needed and where they should be provided, i.e., in a nursing home, a continuing care retirement community (CCRC), or a life care at home (LCAH) program.

Preadmission Testing (PAT)

A type of benefit provided by some health plans designed to encourage members to obtain needed diagnostic services on an ambulatory basis just prior to a non-emergency hospital admission in order to reduce hospital length of stay (LOS).

Preferred Provider

See also:
Participating Provider; Preferred Provider Organization (PPO)

Any physician, hospital or other health care provider who contracts with a particular managed care plan, such as a PPO, to provide health services to persons covered by the plan. Preferred providers may be, but are not necessarily, paid on a fee-for-service basis. Also called a *participating provider*.

Preferred Provider Organization (PPO)

See also:
Free Choice;
Managed Care Plan;
Preferred Provider

A type of *managed care plan* which contracts with independent providers (hospitals, physicians, ancillary providers) for negotiated discounted fees for services provided to plan members. The PPO's network of *preferred providers* is usually limited in size. Unlike an HMO, a PPO is not a prepaid plan, but does use some utilization management techniques. Patients usually have *free choice* of providers but have a financial incentive (e.g., reduced copayments, lower deductibles) to use *participating providers*. PPO arrangements can be either insured or self-funded. An insurer-sponsored PPO combines an extensive network of providers, utilization management programs, administrative services, and health care insurance in one package. A self-funded PPO generally excludes administrative and insurance services from the plan package. However, employers can purchase these services separately.

Prefiling of Fees

See also:
Customary Charge;
Usual, Customary, and Reasonable (UCR)

The process whereby a participating provider submits its usual fees to a managed care plan for the purpose of establishing a *usual, customary, and reasonable (UCR)* range of fees in the geographical area where the participating provider practices.

Premium

See also:
Actuarial Assumptions; Risk Load

A prospectively determined fixed rate which a health plan subscriber pays in periodic amounts per time period (usually per year) for covered services in order to keep an insurance policy in force. The dollar amount of the premium is related to the *actuarial* value of the benefits provided by the policy, plus a "loading" factor (i.e., *risk load*) to cover administrative costs and profit. Premiums are paid for coverage whether the benefits are actually used or not, as opposed to copayments and deductibles, which are paid only if benefits are actually used. Generally, a health plan will have one premium rate for single subscribers and a higher rate for subscribers with dependents.

Premium-Only Plan (POP)

See also:
Cost Sharing Techniques; Flexible Benefit Plan (Flex Plan)

A type of *flexible benefit plan (flex plan)* in which employees are allowed to pay health insurance premiums with pre-tax dollars through salary reductions. Employees' take-home pay is larger and employer payroll taxes are smaller if the rate of the employee contribution remains the same. A POP can be an attractive technique for sharing costs with employees because it requires minimal start-up costs, limited documentation and administrative paperwork, and no restructuring of the underlying benefits.

Prepaid Group Practice Plan

See also:
Foundation for Medical Care (FMC); Group Practice

A type of health plan in which a defined set of services are provided by three or more participating physicians to an enrolled group of persons for a fixed, periodic payment made in advance by or on behalf of each covered person or family. If a health insurance carrier is involved, the term refers to a contract to pay in advance for the full range of services to which the insured is entitled under the terms of the health insurance contract. Such a plan is a form of HMO. Sometimes called a *Medical Foundation* or a *Foundation for Medical Care (FMC).*

Prescription Drug

See also:
Over-the-Counter Drug (OTC)

A drug which has been approved by the Food and Drug Administration (FDA) and, under federal or state law, can be dispensed only by a prescription order from a duly licensed physician (as opposed to an *over-the- counter drug,* which can be purchased directly, without restriction, by consumers). Prescription drugs must bear the label: "Caution: federal law prohibits dispensing without a prescription." Also called a *legend drug.*

P

Prescription Drug Plan

See also:
Drug Formulary; Generic Substitution Program; Mail Order Pharmacy; Prescription Drug

A provision in some health plans which allows members to obtain *prescription drugs* without incurring potentially large out-of-pocket expenses. Different types of outpatient prescription drug benefit plans are available. The most popular are discount plans, *generic substitution programs,* closed panel pharmacy networks, *mail order pharmacies*, and *drug formularies.*

Prevailing Fee

See also:
Prefiling of Fees;
Usual, Customary and Reasonable (UCR)

A fee that falls within the range of fees most frequently charged by providers in a given locality for a particular medical service or procedure. Often, an insurance carrier will consider the prevailing fee as the basis for reimbursement to the provider for services rendered to the insured.

Preventive Care

See also:
Primary Care;
Wellness Program

Comprehensive health care (mostly *primary care*), which emphasizes priorities for prevention, early detection, and early treatment of disease or its consequences. Preventive care usually includes routine physical examinations, immunizations, and *wellness programs.*

Primary Care

See also:
Primary Care Physician / Practitioner (PCP);
Secondary Care;
Tertiary Care

Basic, or first-level, general health care traditionally provided by *primary care physicians (PCP)*, including family practice physicians, pediatricians, internists, and sometimes obstetric/gynecologic (OBGYN) physician specialists. Generally, primary care is provided on an outpatient basis in contrast to *secondary* and *tertiary care,* which involve more complex services and procedures, and inpatient care.

Primary Care Network (PCN)

See also:
Primary Care Physician / Practitioner (PCP)

A group of *primary care physicians (PCP)* who have joined together to share the risk of providing care to members of a managed care plan. The PCP in a primary care network (PCN) is accountable for the total health care services of a plan member, including referrals to specialists, supervision of the specialists' care, and hospitalization, if necessary. Participating PCPs" services are covered by a monthly capitation payment to the PCN, which eliminates the need for claims filing, claims processing, and collection.

Primary Care Physician/ Practitioner (PCP)

See also:
Gatekeeper;
Primary Care Network (PCN)

A physician (general or family practitioner, internist, pediatrician, and sometimes obstetrician/gynecologist), nurse practitioner (NP), or physician's assistant (PA). Managed care plans use PCPs to serve as the initial screening, testing, treatment, and referral source for plan members. Generally, the PCP assumes continuing responsibility for the overall course of treatment of the member. PCPs often acts as *gatekeepers* for managed care plans, determining if a patient's illness requires more costly, specialized treatments by specialists, and/or hospital care.

Primary Payer

See also:
Coordination of Benefits (COB);
Duplication of Benefits

Under *coordination of benefit (COB)* rules, the primary payer is the insurance carrier or the managed care plan that is obligated to pay eligible expenses without consideration of coverage by any other health plan. For example, Medicare is the primary payer with respect to Medicaid. Thus, for a beneficiary who is eligible under both programs, Medicaid (the secondary payer) pays only for benefits not covered under Medicare (the primary payer).

Principal Diagnosis

See also:
Comorbidity;
Diagnosis

The health condition that has been determined, after evaluation, to be chiefly responsible for the admission of the patient to a hospital for inpatient care or for treatment in an ambulatory care setting.

Principal Sum

An amount of money payable in one lump sum to the health plan beneficiary in the event of accidental death or, in some cases, accidental dismemberment.

Prior Authorization

See also:
Authorization;
Out-of-Network Services (OON);
Preadmission Certification

A requirement of some managed care plans that a provider must justify the need for delivering a particular service or medication to a plan member and obtain approval from the plan before actually providing the service as a condition of reimbursement. *Prior authorization* also refers to a document prepared by the primary care physician and approved by the plan's medical director or his/her designee, which authorizes a plan member to receive *out-of-network services* from a non-participatory provider. Without this prior authorization, the service or medication is not covered, nor is it reimbursed. Prior authorization is intended to serve as a cost control mechanism, similar to a purchase order, which validates that the authorized out-of-network review or service is needed.

Priority Setting

See also:
Formal Grievance Procedure

In claims processing, refers to a process of determining the rank order of identified problems for resolution, based on the benefits that would be derived, as well as the risks realized should the problem go unresolved. Priority setting usually occurs during claims disputes and *formal grievance procedures.*

Private Insurer/ Carrier

See also:
Blue Cross/Blue Shield Plans (BC/BS);
Carrier

Usually refers to a non-profit insurance company, such as *Blue Cross and Blue Shield Plans (BC/BS).*

Producer Price Index-Hospital (PPI-H)

See also:
Consumer Price Index (CPI)

A new national indicator of hospital price changes which was recently instituted by the Department of Labor's Bureau of Labor Statistics (February 12, 1993). The hospital component of the producer price index (PPI-H) measures the change in net prices charged by hospitals over time to patients for a hypothetical hospital visit and all of the services provided during that one visit. The PPI-H reflects all charges, including discounts and managed care contracts, as well as Medicare, Medicaid, and rural hospital payments, but does not include bad debt. The seasonally adjusted monthly index is compared with the PPI-H base figure of 100 for December, 1992. By contrast, the medical and hospital components of the other national barometer, the *consumer price index (CPI),* which is used to measure retail price changes over time, measure only out-of-pocket expenditures by consumers, and do not include expenditures from any other sources, such as Medicare and Medicaid.

Productivity

See also:
Performance Standards

A performance indicator which measures the volume of care delivered per given time period, when quality and/or outcome are held constant. For example, a physician who sees six patients per hour is considered more "productive" than one who sees four per hour, if the patients have similar conditions, receive necessary and appropriate care, and have similar outcomes.

Professional Activities Survey (PAS)

A national comparative data reporting program for hospitals. Hospitals purchase the PAS from the Commission on Professional and Hospital Activities (CPHA), a non-profit computer center in Ann Arbor, MI. Information enters the system via the discharge abstract completed by the hospital on every discharged patient. Patient information is returned to the hospital in a series of periodic reports, which compare the hospital's average length of stay (ALOS), number and types of tests used, and autopsy rates for given diagnostic conditions with those of other hospitals of similar size and services. The PAS also is used by many managed care organizations to assist in provider evaluations and plan management.

Professional Liability Insurance (PLI)

See also:
Malpractice Insurance; Medical Negligence

A type of insurance that physicians and other practitioners purchase to help protect themselves from the financial risks associated with claims of medical negligence and malpractice claims and awards. Also called *malpractice insurance.*

Professional Standards Review Organization (PSRO)

See also:
Peer Review Organization (PRO); Tax Equity and Fiscal Responsibility Act of 1982 (TEFRA)

A government-mandated organization (now defunct) composed of local practicing physicians. PSROs contracted with HCFA to review health care services covered under Medicare, Medicaid, and Maternal and Infant Care (MIC) programs. The goal was to confirm that services paid for under these programs was medically necessary, appropriate, and consistent with professionally recognized standards of quality. The federal requirement for establishing PSROs was added to the Social Security Act in 1972. The program was repealed by the *Tax Equity and Fiscal Responsibility Act of 1982 (TEFRA)* and PSROs were replaced by *Peer Review Organizations (PRO).*

Profile Analysis

See also:
Peer Review Organization (PRO); Practice Pattern; Provider Profiling

An examination of a *Peer Review Organization's (PRO)* data or other regional data to identify problems or potential problems in the delivery of health care services. A profile analysis uses statistical summaries of the *practice patterns* of an individual physician, a specific hospital, or the medical experience of a specific population.

Proration

See also:
Duplication of Benefits; Premium

The adjustment of benefits paid due to a mistake in the amount of *premium* paid or the existence of other insurance covering the same accident or disability (i.e., *duplication of benefits*).

Prospective Payment Assessment Commission (ProPAC)

See also:
Medicare; Prospective Payment System (PPS)

A government agency established under the Social Security Act Amendments of 1983 to advise Congress and the Department of Health and Human Services regarding maintaining and updating *Medicare* payments to hospitals and other provider facilities. Because ProPAC is an appointed advisory body, it has no regulatory or appeals authority. ProPAC's responsibilities include Medicare inpatient and outpatient hospital payment policies, prospective payment policies for skilled nursing facilities and home health services, and payment for services furnished in end stage renal disease (ESRD) facilities. ProPAC also is required to examine uncompensated care and Medicaid payments, and their relationship to the financial condition of hospitals.
Address: ProPAC, 300 7th Street, SW, Suite 301-B, Washington, DC 20024
Phone: (202) 401-8986; Fax: (202) 401-8739

P

Prospective Payment System (PPS)

See also:
Medicare Part A; Prospective Rating; Prospective Reimbursement

A term applied to any reimbursement system that pays in advance (i.e., "prospectively") rather than on the basis of charges. Generally, payment rates are established in advance by the managed care plan for the coming year. Providers are then paid these amounts regardless of the costs that they actually incur. The PPS system is designed to introduce constraints on cost increases by setting limits on amounts that will be paid during a future period. PPS is used most often to refer to hospital reimbursement based on DRGs, as in the *Medicare Part* A program.

Prospective Rating

See also:
Experience Rating; Trend Factor

A method of setting premium rates at the beginning of the plan year based on a formula that uses historical experience and *trend factors*. Under the prospective rating system, if the managed care plan does better than expected (i.e., uses fewer claim dollars than anticipated when the premium was initially set), the plan or insurer keeps the difference. If utilization experience is worse than expected, the plan or insurer must cover the difference. Since the prospectively set premium reflects past utilization experience and managed care plans usually are able to improve upon historical (often "unmanaged") experience through utilization management techniques, many employers prefer prospective rating so that they can benefit faster from utilization controls. Also known as *experience rating.*

Prospective Reimbursement

See also:
Prospective Payment System (PPS); Prospective Rating; Retrospective Reimbursement

A method of paying providers for a defined period (usually one year) according to amounts or rates of payment established in advance. The prospective reimbursement system (also called the *prospective payment system*) introduces constraints on cost increases by setting limits on amounts that will be paid during a future period. It also provides incentives for improved efficiency by sharing savings with providers that perform at lower than anticipated costs. In other words, the provider gets to keep the difference if its costs are less than the plan's fixed payment price for a service. However, the provider must absorb any losses if its costs are above the fixed price. (Contrast with *retrospective reimbursement.*)

Prospective Review

See also:
Preadmission Certification; Utilization Review (UR)

A review by a *utilization review (UR)* committee of a proposed schedule of treatment prior to a plan member's admission to a hospital or treatment in an ambulatory care center. The purpose of the prospective review is to ensure the appropriateness and medical necessity of the proposed level of care. The prospective review can cover patient care, discharge plans, as well as any policies or procedures that specify how care will be provided. Also called *preadmission certification.*

P

Provider

See also:
Provider Panel

Refers to any individual or organization that provides health care services. Providers may be physicians, hospitals, physical therapists, medical equipment suppliers, pharmacies, etc.

Provider Panel

See also:
Closed Panel; Open Panel; Provider

A group of *providers* who have contracted with a managed care plan to provide medical services to plan members. A provider panel may be an *open panel*, as in an IPA model HMO, or a *closed panel*, as in a staff, group, or network model HMO.

Provider Profiling

See also:
Practice Pattern; Profile Analysis

The process of collecting and analyzing data linked to the activities of providers (usually physicians) in order to develop provider-specific profiles of practice behavior. Types of provider-related data that might be examined include: health care resource consumption, outcomes, claims data, credentialing data, etc. Managed care organizations may use provider profiling for selecting and recruiting providers for networks, identifying specialists for referrals, detecting fraud and abuse, and modifying providers' *practice patterns*.

Psychographics

See also:
Demographics

The study of subjective characteristics of populations, such as attitudes, perceptions, opinions, and preferences, regarding what people know, believe, and feel about themselves and their health, about health services and the health system, and about specific providers and health plans. Psychographic information is useful for forecasting how people will use specific services or providers. Some researchers consider psychographic factors better discriminators for who is likely to use specific services than *demographic* factors.

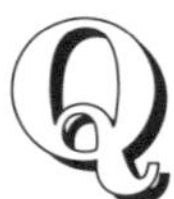

Qualified Impairment Insurance

See also:
Substandard Insurance

A form of special class, or *substandard insurance*, which restricts benefits for an insured person's particular condition.

Qualified Medicare Beneficiary (QMB)

See also:
Beneficiary;
Medicare Part B

A person whose income falls below the federal poverty guidelines and for whom the state must pay the *Medicare Part B* premiums, deductibles, and copayments.

Qualifying Event

See also:
Continuation of Coverage;
COBRA

Refers to an occurrence that entitles a person to choose to continue coverage under *COBRA*. Examples of qualifying events include: termination of employment, reduction of work hours, death of a covered employee, divorce or legal separation, eligibility for Medicare, a dependent's loss of dependent status, loss of coverage due to the employer's filing for bankruptcy, etc.

Quality Assessment

See also:
Pre-established Criteria;
Quality Assurance (QA);
Standards

The measurement phase in a *quality assurance (QA)* program, in which *pre-established criteria* or *standards* for professional performance, with respect to patient, administrative, and support services, are compared against the health care actually provided. The medical record is used as documentation of the care provided.

Q

Quality Assurance (QA)

See also:
Quality Assessment

A formal set activities that measure the kind and degree of excellence of health care services provided. Quality assurance includes both a measurement phase (see *quality assessment*) and corrective actions to remedy any deficiencies identified through the quality assessment process. There are some federal and state guidelines that govern QA programs for HMOs. Many managed care organizations have QA programs for reviewing provider practice patterns and utilization management procedures to ensure that quality of care is being maintained and not sacrificed as a result of a desire to control health care costs.

Quality Improvement Program (QIP)

See also:
Continuous Quality Improvement (CQI); Total Quality Management (TQM)

A formal, ongoing process of identifying problems in health care delivery, testing solutions to those problems, and continually monitoring the solutions for improvement. QIP is a common feature of *total quality management (TQM)* programs. Generally, an organization undertakes QIP to achieve continual improvement in the quality of operations and elimination of waste in all functions of the organization through design and redesign processes. The aim of QIP is elimination of variations or "defects" in health care delivery through elimination of their causes. Sometimes called *Continuous Quality Improvement (CQI).*

Quality Indicator

See also:
Indicator; Quality of Care (QC)

A measure of the degree of excellence of health care actually provided. Selected "quality indicators" of patient outcome, such as mortality and morbidity, health status, length of stay, readmission rate, patient satisfaction, etc., are considered by many groups to be measures of the quality of care. However, there appears to be no consensus at the present time on what constitutes meaningful measures of quality. Nevertheless, most health care experts agree that *quality of care*, or "value," is closely related to patient outcomes and cost. A number of public and private initiatives currently are attempting to define health care quality, identify appropriate quality indicators, and develop standards for measuring quality.

Quality of Care (QC)

See also:
Quality Assurance (QA); Quality Indicator

A desired degree of excellence in the provision of health care. Though quality is a subjective attribute, various characteristics usually associated with the health care delivery process are thought to be determinants of quality. These include: structural adequacy, access and availability, technical abilities of practitioners, practitioner communication skills and attitudes, documentation of services provided, coordination and follow-up, patient commitment and adherence to a therapeutic regimen, patient satisfaction, and clinical outcome.

Quality Review Committee (QRC)

See also:
Peer Review Organization (PRO); Quality Assurance (QA); Quality of Care (QC)

A committee established by a professional organization or institution to assess and/or ensure the quality of care provided to patients. Unlike *peer review organizations (PRO)*, a QRC can function on its own initiative on a broad range of topics relating to health care quality.

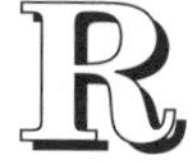

Radiologists, Anaesthesiologists, and Pathologists (RAP)

A category of physician specialists who occasionally, but not always, are included in a managed care plan's network of preferred providers. Since plan members typically do not select these specialists to handle their cases, RAPs usually are not included in a plan's provider network, since it would be inappropriate for the plan to pay preferred or non-preferred benefits for RAP services depending on whether or not the member used a contracted provider. Generally, RAPs are included in a plan's provider network only if the plan can obtain full participation by the RAP physicians in a multispecialty physician group with which the plan contracts.

Rate

See also:
Premium;
Rating Process

The amount of *premium* per enrollment or per risk classification that is paid to an insurance carrier or managed care plan for medical coverage. Premium rates are usually fixed for a year and paid on a monthly basis.

Rate Cells

See also:
HCFA Rate Cell Verification;
Medicare Risk Contract

A set of 122 monthly capitation amounts which HCFA pays HMOs and competitive medical plans (CMPs) having a *Medicare Risk contract* for each Medicare beneficiary. Medicare beneficiaries are grouped in rate cells based on five variables: age, sex, Medicaid eligibility, institutional status, and whether or not a person has both parts of Medicare (Part A for inpatient services and Part B for all other services).

Rate Guarantee

See also:
Consumer Price Index (CPI);
Rate;
Rating Process

In group health plans, monthly premium rates are usually guaranteed to remain fixed for a specified period, usually one year. Generally, the longer the rate guarantee, the higher the premium rate. This is because of the difficulty of projecting the cost of health care in the future. Another reason for setting higher premium rates for longer rate guarantee periods is because of the expectation that health care costs will continue to rise faster than the *consumer price index (CPI).*

Rate-Setting

See also:
National Health Expenditures (NHE)

The process of determining rates to be paid by a government agency to a health care provider based on actual and projected costs of services. For example, rate-setting under proposed national health care reform initiatives would establish cost targets for overall *national health expenditure (NHE)* categories. The NHE budget would be divided into two sectors, Medicare and non-Medicare, with each sector subject to different annual limits on hospital expenditures. Separate limits would be established for physicians' services. This type of rate-setting is designed to involve federal and state governments more directly in achieving cost containment objectives.

Rating Process

See also:
Premium;
Rate

The process of evaluating an individual or group to determine a premium rate based on a rating formula and related to the type of risk the individual or group presents. Key components of a typical rating formula are: age and sex factors, location, type of industry, base capitation factor, plan design, average family size, demographics, and administrative costs.

Reasonable and Customary Charge (R&C)

See also:
Customary Charge;
Usual, Customary, and Reasonable (UCR)

A charge for health care services that is consistent with the going rate or charge within a certain geographical area for identical or similar services. A fee is considered to be "reasonable" if it falls within parameters of the average or commonly charged ("customary") fee for the particular service within that specific community.

Recertification

See also:
Continued Stay Review (CSR)

The process of reviewing and authorizing the medical necessity and appropriateness of continuation of a plan member's stay at a hospital at a particular level of care. Also called *continued stay review (CSR).* The term also may refer to the certification of a provider's continuing education in order to maintain a current license to practice in his/her specialty.

Recidivism Refers to the frequency of the same patient returning to the hospital for inpatient hospitalization or to an outpatient center for repetitive ambulatory care for the same presenting problem(s).

Recipient
See also:
Beneficiary

A person who has been designated by a Medicaid agency as eligible to receive Medicaid benefits. Also can refer to a Medicare *beneficiary*.

Reciprocity An agreement between two or more managed care plans that permits a member of one plan, who is temporarily away from home, to receive treatment from another prepaid plan for illness or injuries that cannot be postponed until the member returns to his/her home service area.

Reconsideration See: **Expedited Appeal**

Recurring Clause A provision in some health insurance policies that specifies a period of time during which the recurrence of a medical condition is considered a continuation of a prior period of disability or hospital confinement rather than a separate episode of illness.

Reference Projection A forecast of expected future activity levels on various types of planning data if no actions are taken to alter current activities and commitments. Reference projections include data on various indicators, such as demographic and environmental factors, financial factors, resources, health service utilization, etc.

Referral

See also:
Referral Specialist;
Self-Referral

A recommendation by a physician and/or managed care plan for a plan member to be evaluated and/or treated by a different physician. The referral physician (i.e., the physician to whom the member is referred) could be another primary care physician or specialist who may or may not be in the plan's network. In a group model HMO, referrals are usually to specialists within the group, unless the group does not have specialists qualified to provide needed services.

Referral Agency

See also:
Employee Assistance Program (EAP);
Referral

An agency or institution to which a plan member is referred for continuing treatment. The referral may be made by a primary care physician, an employee assistance program (EAP), the employee benefit plan, or by another health care institution. For example, an EAP may refer an employee with a known chemical dependency problem to an appropriate referral agency, such as Alcoholics Anonymous, which offers counseling and other treatment programs.

Referral Specialist

See also:
Referral

A medical or surgical specialist who provides a service to a plan member who has been referred to him/her by a primary care physician or another specialist who may or may not be a participating provider in the patient's managed care plan.

Regional Health Alliance

See also:
American Health Security Act of 1993 (AHSA);
Health Alliance;
Health Insurance Purchasing Cooperative (HIPC);
Managed Competition

Under the proposed *American Health Security Act of 1993 (AHSA),* a large pool of businesses and individuals in a geographical area which purchases health care coverage for enrolled individuals. Regional health alliances would represent the interests of consumers and purchasers of health care services, and assure that all residents in an area who are covered through the alliance receive the nationally guaranteed benefits. They also would be responsible for structuring the market to encourage delivery of high quality, cost-effective care. Each alliance would include among its plan offerings at least one fee-for-service plan. The alliance would establish a fee schedule and providers would not be allowed to charge fees in excess of the allowable charges. Each state would be responsible for establishing and governing one or more regional health alliance to cover residents in every area of the state. Regional health alliances are similar in many ways to the *health insurance purchasing cooperatives (HIPC)* in the Jackson Hole Group's *managed competition* model for health care reform.

Regionalization

See also:
Integrated Delivery System (IDS)

A concept of shared facilities and resources for the maximizing of services. For example, an *integrated delivery system (IDS)* may have several hospitals in a large geographical area or region in its integrated provider network who share certain equipment, such as a mobile lithotriptsy or MRI unit, or the expenses of certain marketing programs, such as a direct mail campaign to residents in the hospitals' respective service areas, or a team of specialists which moves from facility to facility according to a weekly rotation schedule.

Registered Nurse (RN)

A nurse who has graduated from a formal, accredited program of nursing education and has been granted a Registered Nurse (RN) license by the appropriate state authority after passing a licensing examination. Registered nurses are the most highly educated of nurses and tend to have the widest scope of responsibility for all aspects of nursing care.

Rehabilitation

See also:
Total Disability

Refers to the restoration of a totally disabled person to the highest possible level of functional ability. Rehabilitation generally involves the combined and coordinated use of medical, social, educational and vocational measures for training or retraining. Rehabilitation also may refer to a provision in some long-term disability policies which provides for continuation of benefits or other financial assistance while a totally disabled insured person is retraining or attempting to resume productive employment.

Reinstatement

See also:
Lapse

The resumption of coverage under a policy that has *lapsed*.

Reinsurance

See also:
Stop-Loss Reinsurance

A type of insurance purchased by primary insurers (i.e., insurers that provide health care coverage directly to policyholders) from other secondary insurers, called "reinsurers," to protect against part or all of the losses the primary insurer might incur in honoring the claims of its policyholders. In other words, reinsurance is a transaction between and among insurers for the assumption of risk in exchange for a premium. Usually, a primary insurer will "cede" only a portion of its total risk and premium payments to a reinsurer, either as a percentage of total premiums or only for losses above a particular threshold. Reinsurance is used to spread insurable risk, protect assets against excessive claims losses, and increase financial capacity to underwrite coverage beyond what is affordable, given the insurer's level of financial surplus.

Relative Value of Services (RVS)

See also:
Current Procedural Terminology (CPT); Customary Charge; Resource Based Relative Value Scale (RBRVS)

A type of pricing system for physicians' services which assigns relative values to procedures based on a defined standard unit of measure, as defined in the *current procedural terminology (CPT).* RVS units are based on median charges by physicians. Time, skill, and overhead costs required for each service are taken into account, but not the relative cost-effectiveness of the service, relative need or demand for it, or its importance to people's health. RVS allows performance comparisons of medical services in terms reflective of true costs. Physicians often use the RVS system as a guide in establishing fee schedules. Insurers, managed care companies, and the federal government also use the RVS system for determining reimbursement, especially in geographical areas where no*customary charge* is established for a covered service.

Reliability

See also:
Indicator

In research, the precision or consistency with which an *indicator* or measurement can yield identical or highly similar results with repeated testing. Reliability, however, does not ensure that the results are correct or valid, only that they are consistent.

Renal Dialysis Center

See also:
End Stage Renal Disease (ESRD)

A facility that furnishes the full spectrum of diagnostic, therapeutic and rehabilitative services (except renal transplants) required for the care of *end stage renal disease (ESRD)* dialysis patients. Renal dialysis centers may provide the services directly, or indirectly through other facilities in a network.

Renewal

See also:
Lapse;
Reinstatement

Continuance of coverage under a policy beyond its original term by the insurer's acceptance of the premium or a letter of intent to pay the premium for a new policy term.

Representative Sample

A subgroup of individuals whose characteristics are similar in nature and in frequency of occurrence to those of a total population from which the sample is drawn. Representative samples usually are used in managed care research for studying whole populations.

Request for Information (RFI)

See also:
Request for Proposal (RFP)

In seeking a managed care provider for its employees, an employer (or the consultant, broker, agent, etc. representing the employer's interests) sometimes solicits preproposal information from potential provider partners prior to sending out *requests for proposals (RFP).* The RFI helps the employer determine which managed care organizations will receive the RFP.

Request for Proposal (RFP)

See also:
Request for Information (RFI)

A formal solicitation for bids from interested parties for selected services, special projects, or other undertakings. Often, RFPs are issued by employers and government agencies seeking managed care providers. The RFP may be issued directly to prospective provider partners (e.g., hospitals, managed care organizations, specialty providers, etc.), or indirectly through a consultant, broker, or agent. It is sent to a selected list of organizations after a careful assessment of potential candidates. The RFP may ask for financial data, information about claims, the company's experience, a proposed benefit design, and reasons why the organization is best suited for the employer. Sometimes, an employer or consultant will issue a *request for information (RFI)* prior to the RFP in order to gather preproposal information to help it determine which organizations will receive the RFP.

Reserves

See also:
Expected Claims; Incurred But Not Reported (IBNR)

The measure of an insurer's or managed care organization's financial capability to fund liabilities for future claims or cost of health care. For each insured group, insurers estimate the amount of money they will need to fund claims payments for which they will be liable under outstanding insurance policies. The reserve estimate is added to an estimate of claims payments for a contract year in order to arrive at an *expected claims* projection for the group. Estimated reserves have four principal components: 1) reserves for known liabilities not yet paid; 2) reserves for losses *incurred but not reported (IBNR)*; 3) reserves for future benefits; and 4) other reserves for various special purposes, including contingency reserves for unforeseen circumstances.

Residential Care Facility (RCF)

A house or other type of lodging facility with a program that provides shelter, food, laundry, social, and sometimes spiritual support to adults needing such care. A common example is a home for the aged.

Residential Mental Health Program

A treatment program for psychiatric disorders which offers 24-hour care that is less intensive than the care in an inpatient hospital setting. Substance abuse is usually excluded from this type of treatment program.

Residual Disability Benefit

See also:
Lifetime Disability Benefit;
Partial Disability

A provision in an insurance policy which provides benefits in proportion to a reduction of earnings as a result of a covered person's *partial disability*, unlike a *lifetime disability benefit* which replaces lost income as long as the covered person is totally disabled.

Resource Based Relative Value Scale (RBRVS)

See also:
Fee Schedule;
Performance Standards;
Relative Value of Services (RVS)

A fee schedule developed by Harvard researchers for the federal government to provide a more equitable physician reimbursement system for services provided to Medicare beneficiaries. Unlike the *relative value of services (RVS)* system, RBRVS attempts to take into account all the resources–physical, educational, mental, financial–that physicians use in caring for patients. Relative values have been formulated for 2,700 codes, which account for 95% of Medicare- allowed charges. Payment amounts are adjusted for geographical differences in practice costs. In 1992, HCFA began phasing in RBRVS for Medicare reimbursement over a five-year period to establish volume *performance standards* for physicians' services, which will be used for updating Medicare's physician *fee schedule*. Several private insurers (e.g., Blue Cross & Blue Shield) have begun phasing in the RBRVS reimbursement system for selected procedures.

Resource Capacity

See also:
Resources

Refers to the amount, type, and distribution of health services that can be provided by the usable, available resources in a given geographical area.

Resource Costs

See also:
Resources;
Resource Based Relative Value Scale (RBRVS)

Refers to the costs of the "inputs" needed to provide a service or procedure by an efficient provider. Resource costs are used for establishing the *resource based relative value scale (RBRVS),* and include both the opportunity costs of the physician's own time and effort and the costs of non-physician inputs. Physicians' efforts in supervising and managing quality control activities, however, are not reflected in resource input costs used to calculate RBRVS fees.

Resources

See also:
Medical Supplies;
Resource Costs

In the delivery of health care services, resources generally refer to the facilities, labor force, medical supplies, money, knowledge, and other sources of support needed to accomplish a set of program objectives.

Retention

See also:
Administrative Costs

Refers to the portion of the cost of a health benefit program that is retained by the insurance carrier or managed care plan to cover internal costs, such as taxes, claims processing, printing, supplies, and all other expenses and risk factors, or to return a profit. Also called *administrative costs.*

Retiree Medical Plans

Refers to group-sponsored or employer-sponsored medical plans for retirees that are integrated with Medicare benefits but are not *Medicare Supplement Policies.*

Retrospective Premium

See also:
Premium;
Retention

An arrangement between an insurer and a policyholder whereby the insured agrees to pay an additional premium at the end of the contract year if claims and *retention* (i.e., administrative costs) exceed the total paid premiums.

Retrospective Rate Derivation (Retro)

See also:
Loss Ratio;
Risk Sharing

A provision in some group insurance policies which requires some *risk sharing* with the employer. For example, the employer may be financially liable for a prenegotiated percentage of its employees' health care costs in excess of total premium dollars paid by the employer during the contract year. The insurer agrees to collect less than the standard premium during the year, but if the actual *loss ratio* exceeds the loss ratio agreed upon at the beginning of the year plus the total premium paid, the employer must make up the difference. Usually there is a maximum cap to the additional premium for which the employer is liable. Likewise, the insurance carrier may be required to refund to the employer a percentage of premium paid if actual health costs of the insured group are less than the premium dollars paid during the contract year.

R

Retrospective Reimbursement

See also:
Prospective Reimbursement

A payment to a provider by a third party payor for costs or charges actually incurred by a plan member in a previous time period. Also called *cost-based* or *fee-for-service reimbursement*. (Contrast with *prospective reimbursement*.)

Revenue Codes

See also:
Uniform Billing Code of 1992 (UB-92)

Coded descriptions of an institution's cost centers found on the summary sheet of the standard billing form, called the *UB-92* form. Physical therapy, surgery, room and board, for example, have specific revenue codes. (In 1993, the UB-82 form was replaced by a UB-92 form. However, in many health care organizations, this standard billing form is still called the UB-82 form.)

Rider

A legal document which modifies or amends the coverage under an insurance policy. For example, a rider may increase or decrease benefits, waive the condition of coverage, or in any other way amend the original contract.

Risk

See also:
Capitation;
Risk Management;
Risk Sharing

Potential financial liability, particularly as it pertains to who or what is legally responsible for that liability. With insurance, risk is limited by the policy's dollar limitations. Providers (e.g., hospitals and physicians) bear risk if they are paid a fixed amount for services rendered to members of a managed care plan. For example, providers that are reimbursed on a capitated basis share the financial risk of the potential cost of services and resources utilized in the course of a patient's treatment. If the cost of care exceeds the capitated amount of reimbursement received, the provider absorbs the excess costs. If the cost of provided services is less than the capitated payment, the provider retains the excess revenue.

Risk Adjustment

See also:
American Health Security Act of 1993 (AHSA);
National Health Board (NHB);
Regional Health Alliance;
Risk

Under the proposed *American Health Security Act of 1993 (AHSA)*, a *regional health alliance (RHA)* would be permitted to adjust premium payments to health plans to reflect the level of risk assumed for plan enrollees compared to the average population in the geographical area served by the RHA. The risk adjustment mechanism would take into account factors such as age, gender, health status, and services to disadvantaged populations. The risk adjustment system would be established by the *National Health Board (NHB)* nine months before the date on which states first enroll consumers in RHAs. RHAs would be required to use the risk adjustment system unless an alliance obtains a waiver from the NHB.

Risk Analysis

See also:
Actuary;
Risk

The process of evaluating the expected costs of medical care for a group seeking health care benefits under a particular health plan. Risk analysis helps managed care organizations and insurers determine what products, benefit levels, and prices to offer in order to best meet the needs of both the group and the plan.

Risk and Insurance Management Society, Inc. (RIMS)

A professional association for employee benefits managers of large corporations, non-profit and public sector institutions, and government agencies. RIMS offers educational courses, conferences and seminars, monitors regulatory and legislative developments, and represents members' positions concerning reform issues that affect the stability of the risk management and 770
employee benefits environment. RIMS also conducts research on emerging trends and publishes periodicals, books, and other resources. RIMS' Associate in Risk Management Program professional credentialing program is offered in conjunction with the Insurance Institute of America.
Address: RIMS, 205 East 42nd St., 15th Floor,
New York, NY 10017
Phone: (212) 286-9292; Fax: (212) 986-9716

Risk Charge

See also:
Surplus

The portion of a premium that is used to generate or replenish the surpluses that an insurance carrier is required to develop in order to offset potential losses under its policies. Profits, if any, on the sale of insurance are also taken from the risk charges.

Risk Contract

See: **Medicare Risk Contract**

Risk Control Insurance

See: **Reinsurance** and **Stop-Loss Reinsurance**

R

Risk Factors

See also:
Risk Analysis;
Risk Load

Refers to certain conditions that influence a person's health. Generally, risk factors are capable of provoking ill health. Risk factors include inherited or acquired biological conditions, environmental and occupational hazards, and behavioral risk factors.

Risk Load

See also:
Rating Process;
Risk Factor

A weighting factor used by insurance carriers and managed care plans to calculate premium rates for each enrolled group. The risk load is factored into the premium rate to offset some adverse parameter in the group.

Risk Management

See also:
Risk

A comprehensive program of activities to identify, evaluate, and take corrective action against *risks* that may lead to patient or employee injury, and property loss or damage with resulting financial loss or legal liability.

Risk Pool

See also:
Capitation;
Physician Contingency Reserve (PCR);
Withhold

A pool of funds established by a managed care plan (typically an HMO) in a risk sharing arrangement (i.e., *capitation*) with providers. Funds are derived from withholding a portion of provider fees or capitation payments in order to create a financial reserve to cover unanticipated utilization of services. Any funds left over at the end of a period (usually one year), are distributed among the providers.

Risk Sharing

See also:
Capitation

A method by which premiums and costs of medical services are shared by both the managed care plan's sponsor and plan members. Risk sharing also refers to shared financial liability between a managed care plan and a provider for health services delivered to plan members. For example, in a *capitation* arrangement, the managed care plan pays providers in its network a fixed amount for services rendered to a plan member regardless of the cost, level, or extent of the services. If the cost of services is less than the capitated reimbursement amount, the provider comes out ahead, and vice versa.

Robert Wood Johnson Foundation (RWJF)

A national health philanthropy which designs, funds, and evaluates health services and health policy research projects which support the organization's four main goals: 1) improving access for Americans of all ages to basic health care; 2) improving service systems for people with chronic health conditions; 3) promoting health and preventing disease by reducing harm caused by substance abuse; and 4) addressing the problem of rising health care costs. The RWJF publishes a quarterly newsletter, Advances, sponsors educational forums, and offers educational materials produced by RWJF-funded projects to the public.
Address: RWJF, College Road, P.O. Box 2316, Princeton, NJ 08543-2316
Phone: (609) 452-8701

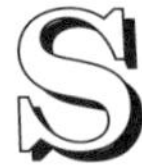

Safe Harbor Regulations

See also:
Hospital-Physician Alliance (HPA); Medicare / Medicaid Fraud and Abuse Statute

A set of federal regulations which clarify and ease the restrictions of the *Medicare / Medicaid Fraud & Abuse Statute*. Safe harbor regulations specify certain types of provider payment arrangements that are not subject to criminal prosecution or civil sanctions, such as the sale of a practice from one provider to another, payments by hospitals to bona fide employees enabling a hospital to pay its employed physicians. Safe harbor regulations have important implications regarding *hospital-physician alliances* and physician recruiting practices. With fewer regulatory barriers, hospitals and physicians are more likely to collaborate with one another.

Sanction

A reprimand of a participating provider by a managed care plan for any number of reasons. Managed care plans likewise can incur state or federal sanctions.

Scheduled Plan

See also:
Fee Schedule; Table of Allowances

A type of health plan (typically fee-for-service insurance) which provides specific allowances for each covered service. The list of fees is called the *table of allowances*. The sum of all the allowances represents the total financial obligation of the plan for payment of covered health care services for the plan member. Payments may be made either to enrollees or on assignment directly to the provider.

Screening

See also:
Pre-established Criteria

In claims review, the process of identifying claims that are not covered or are deficient in some respect. In utilization management, screening refers to the initial process of separating from a group those cases that do not conform to pre-established criteria or quality guidelines, and thus require additional investigation.

Second Surgical Opinion (SSO)

See also:
Utilization Management (UM)

A *utilization management* technique whereby a plan member is encouraged or required to obtain an additional medical opinion(s) from other specialists prior to making a decision about surgical procedures. Second surgical opinion (SSO) programs can be voluntary or mandatory. In a voluntary program, the plan member is informed that a second opinion is covered if the member wishes to obtain one. Under a mandatory program, reimbursement is reduced if a second opinion is not received prior to surgery. A list of surgical procedures that are subject to SSO is usually developed jointly by the managed care plan and medical specialists who generally do not have first contact with the patient.

Secondary Care

See also:
Primary Care;
Tertiary Care

Refers to "second level" medical services usually provided by medical specialists, such as cardiologists, urologists, and dermatologists, who generally do not have first contact with patients. Generally, secondary care involves inpatient hospitalization which does not require highly specialized, complex medical services or equipment. Secondary care may also include ambulatory surgery services, such as routine surgery for gall stones, hernia repair, etc.

Secondary Coverage

See also:
Coordination of Benefits (COB);
Duplication of Benefits

In cases where *duplication of benefits* exist, secondary coverage refers to the health plan that is responsible for payment of any eligible charges that are not covered by the primary coverage.

Section 125 Plan

See also:
Cafeteria Plan;
Flexible Benefit Plan (Flex Plan)

Refers to a type of *flexible benefit plan*. The term derives from the section in the Internal Revenue Code which defines such plans (legally known as *cafeteria plans*) and stipulates that employee contributions to Section 125 plans may be made with pretax dollars.

Selective Contracting

See also:
Any Willing Provider;
Third Party Payor

Negotiation by third party payors of a limited number of contracts with physicians, other health care professionals, and provider facilities in a given service area. Plan members receiving treatment from these "selected" providers are offered preferential benefits.

Self-Administered Plan

See also:
Employee Benefits Information System (EBIS);
Self-Funded Plan

A health plan (typically, a *self-funded plan*) which is administered by the employer rather than an intermediate insurance carrier. The employer maintains all records concerning its employees covered under the group plan. Some of the benefits may be insured or subcontracted, while others may be self-funded.

Self-Funded Plan

See also:
Administrative Services Only Contract (ASO); Employee Retirement Income Security Act (ERISA); Self-Administered Plan; Third Party Administrator (TPA)

A health care program in which employers (usually large companies with 500 or more employees) fund employee benefits plans from their own resources and directly pay claims instead of purchasing group insurance. In other words, an employer that self-funds covers specified health care costs of its own employees by rather than insuring them. Self-funded plans may be *self-administered*, or the employer may contract with a *third party administrator (TPA)* for *administrative services only (ASO)*. Self-funded employers contract with managed care organizations or directly with providers for health care services for their employees. They may limit their liability with stop-loss insurance on an aggregate and/or individual basis. Self-funding employers are exempted by *ERISA* from state insurance laws, state-mandated requirements for employer health benefit programs, state taxes on insurance premiums, and participation in state risk pools or uncompensated care plans. Also known as *self-insurance*.

Self-Insurance

See: **Self-Funded Plan**

Self-Insurance Institute of America, Inc. (SIIA)

See also:
Self-Funded Plan

A national trade association for the three principal entities of the self-insurance industry–employers, third party administrators (TPA), and reinsurance companies. SIIA's goal is to improve the quality and efficiency of *self-funded plans* and enhance public acceptance of this viable alternative to conventional insurance. SIAA activities include: educational and training programs, publications, and representation of members' concerns in federal legislative and regulatory areas through a political action program.
Address: SIIA, P.O. Box 15466, Santa Ana, CA 92705
Phone: (714) 261-2553; Fax: (714) 261-2594

Self-Pay Option

See also:
COBRA

The opportunity to receive health care benefits offered under some employer-sponsored plans to laid-off workers or employees who work insufficient hours to maintain eligibility for health benefits. Premiums are paid directly by the individual. This arrangement enables the enrollee to avoid lapses in coverage. Often, the self-pay premium does not cover the costs of carrying such individuals, and represents a partial subsidy by the group health plan.

Self-Referral

See also:
Medicare / Medicaid Fraud and Abuse Statute

Arrangements made by the patient rather than the provider for health care services beyond primary care. HMOs usually specify the types of services or specialists to which a patient may self-refer. The term also applies to physician self-referrals, whereby a physician refers patients to facilities in which the physician has an ownership interest. Federal legislation is pending for an across-the-board ban on all physician self-referrals. Currently, the Medicare/ Medicaid Fraud and Abuse Statute (also called the *anti-kickback statute)* prohibits physicians from accepting payments (i.e., "kickbacks") from facilities which are intended to induce the physicians to refer Medicare and Medicaid business to those facilities. The statute also makes profit distributions from joint ventures illegal when they are intended to influence a physician judgment in self-referring Medicare or Medicaid patients to facilities in which the physician is are investor.

Senior Citizen Policies

See also:
Medicare Supplement Policy;
MediGap Insurance

Health insurance contracts covering persons 65 years of age or older. In most cases, these policies supplement the beneficiary's Medicare coverage. Also known as *MediGap Insurance* or *Medicare Supplement Policy*.

S

Service Area

See also:
Catchment Area;
Certificate of Authority (COA);
In-Area Services

The geographical market served by a managed care plan or health care system as approved by the state regulatory agencies and/or as detailed in the *certificate of authority (COA)* for HMOs. Except in bona fide emergencies, enrollees are required to seek care from participating providers who generally are located within the managed care plan's service area.

Service Assessment Program (SAP)

Internal audits conducted by a managed care organization for the purpose of reviewing the accuracy and timeliness of various operations, such as claims payment, enrollment data entry, provider database data entry, etc.

Service Intensity

See also:
Service Intensity Weights (SIW)

Refers to the levels or quantities of services provided to patients in a hospital. Intensity can be expressed in terms of a weighted index of services provided, called a *service intensity weight (SIW),* or in terms of a set of statistics indicating the average number of laboratory tests, surgical procedures, x-rays, and other services provided per patient or per patient day. Service intensity is a function of the type of service and its case mix.

Service Intensity Weights (SIW)

See also:
Service Intensity

A weighting system used by hospitals and managed care organizations to establish the relative quantities of services (i.e., *service intensity*) provided for various DRGs.

Severity of Illness Index

See also:
Outcomes;
Severity-Adjusted Clinical Outcome

A classification system used by many hospitals and managed care organizations to evaluate patient *outcomes* as indicators of the quality of care provided to plan members. The severity of ilness index is based on five factors: age of patient, physiological systems involved in the illness, stage of disease, complications, and patient's response to therapy.

Severity-Adjusted Clinical Outcome

See also:
Outcomes; Outcomes Measurement; Severity of Illness Index

A measure of health care quality which considers the severity of a patient's illness, using the *severity of illness index* in the analysis of the end results of care. Severity-adjusted clinical outcomes include disability, functional status, mortality, morbidity, recovery, and patient satisfaction, adjusted for age, physiological systems involved in the illness, stage of disease, complications, and a patient's response to therapy. These are factored into *outcomes measurements* to provide a more realistic indication of quality of care.

Shadow Pricing

The practice of setting premium rates at a level just below a competitor's rates, whether or not those rates can be justified. This practice is considered unethical and may even be illegal if the premium rates could actually be lower than the "shadow price" but are set higher in order to maximize profits.

Short-Term Disability Income Insurance

A type of insurance contract which provides employment pay benefits to a covered disabled person as long as he/she remains disabled up to a specified period of time, not exceeding two years.

Sickness

See also:
Health Status

In managed care terms, sickness is synonymous with physical illness, disease, or pregnancy, but usually does not include mental illness.

Similarly-Sized Subscriber Group (SSSG)

See also:
Federal Employees Health Benefit Program (FEHBP)

A rating requirement enacted by the Office of Personnel Management for community rated managed care plans to ensure that rates charged to the *Federal Employees Health Benefit Program (FEHBP)* are no greater than rates quoted by the contractor for similarly sized subscriber groups (SSSG). FEHBP regulations defineSSSGs as a contractor's two employer groups whose total number of subscribers are closest in size to FEHBP's enrollment, purchase the same benefits package as offered to federal employees, and are renewed during the plan's fiscal year.

Simplified Payment Method

See also:
Bundled Billing; Coronary Artery Bypass Graft Project (CABG)

An all-inclusive billing method used by providers participating in a Medicare demonstration project for *coronary artery bypass graft (CABG)* surgery. In the simplified payment method, fees for all hospital and physician services associated with the bypass surgery are bundled into a single, package bill, which is submitted to HCFA for payment. Medicare pays a lump sum per CABG case, ranging from $21,092 to $35,182, depending on the hospital and the procedure's complexity. Patients do not receive any bills from the providers. The objective is to control costs and improve quality by compelling physicans and hospitals to share in the financial risks associated with the medical procedure. Also called *bundled billing*.

S

Sixth Omnibus Reconciliation Act (SOBRA)

See: **Omnibus Reconciliation Act (OBRA)**

Skilled Nursing Facility (SNF)

See also:
Nursing Home

A facility, either free-standing or part of a hospital, with a professionally trained staff that provides medical treatment, continuous nursing, rehabilitation, and various other health and social services to patients who are not in an acute phase of illness, but who require skilled care on an inpatient basis in lieu of hospital inpatient services. SNFs must be certified by Medicare and meet specific qualifications, including 24-hour nursing coverage, availability of physical, occupational and speech therapies, and other requirements.

Sliding Fee Scale

A form of payment for medical services in which charges are made according to the patient's income or ability to pay. In a sliding fee scale arrangement, low income patients typically pay less than high income patients for the same services.

Social Security Freeze

A provision in some long-term disability insurance policies which ensures that the offset from benefits paid by Social Security will not be changed regardless of subsequent changes in the Social Security law.

S

Society for Healthcare Planning and Marketing (SHPM)

See also:
American Hospital Association (AHA); Healthcare Provider Networks Section (HPNS)

A professional membership group of the *American Hospital Association (AHA)* serving the needs of health care planning and marketing executives. SHPM offers educational programs on strategic planning, marketing, physician services, sales, and managed care. It also provides access to the AHA's information resources and serves as an information clearinghouse. A newly formed (in 1992) subgroup, the *Healthcare Provider Networks Section (HPNS),* serves the professional interests of managed care executives. SHPM sponsors an annual Managed Care Forum to meet the educational needs of HPNS members.
Address: SHPM, 840 N. Lake Shore Drive
Chicago, IL 60611
Phone: (312) 280-6086; Fax: (312) 280-6252

Society of Professional Benefit Administrators (SPBA)

See also:
Third Party Administrator (TPA)

A national association of about 450 independent *third party administrator* (TPA) firms that manage clients' employee benefit plans. Members' clients include small businesses, large corporations, unions, and association-sponsored plans in every industry and profession. SPBA provides leadership in cost-containment efforts, cost-efficient administration techniques for pension and health benefit plans, as well as understanding of complex government compliance requirements.
Address: SPBA, Two Wisconsin Circle, Suite 670, Chevy Chase, MD 20815
Phone: (301) 718-7722; Fax: (301) 718-9440

Special Risk Insurance

A type of insurance coverage for risks or hazards of a special or unusual nature. These must be specified in the insurance contract.

Specialist

See also:
Specialty Board

Usually refers to a physician, but also may refer to a dentist or other health professional, who voluntarily limits practice to a certain branch of medicine related to specific services or procedures (e.g., surgery, radiology, etc), certain age categories of patients (e.g., pediatrics, geriatrics), specific body systems (e.g., dermatology, cardiology), certain types of diseases (e.g., psychiatry, allergy, or periodontics). Specialists have had special education and training related to their respective practices, and may or may not be certified as specialists by the related specialty board.

Specialty Board

See also:
Board Certified; Certification; Specialist

Medical administrative bodies that regulate specialty and subspecialty fields of medicine, surgery, and dental practice by maintaining quality of care and board recognition of physicians and dentists. The standards for certification relate to length and type of training and experience, and include written and oral examination of applicants for specialty certification.

Specialty Differential

See also:
Specialist

The difference in the relative value or amount of money paid for the same service when performed by different medical *specialists*. For example, a specialty differential may exist between what a specialist in a rural community charges for a certain procedure and what his/her counterpart in a major metropolitan area charges for the same procedure.

Specialty Hospital

See also:
General Hospital; Specialty Network

A medical facility with inpatient beds and medical services for providing diagnosis and treatment of special medical conditions, such as mental disease, chemical dependency, spinal or head injury, etc. Specialty hospitals include: transitional care hospitals, psychiatric hospitals, rehabilitation hospitals, organ transplant centers, and heart transplant centers. (Contrast with *general hospital*.)

Specialty Network

See also:
Bundled Billing; Carve-Out Service; Specialty Hospital

A type of quality-focused managed care network in which certain types of services, such as organ transplants, spinal and head injury care, specialized orthopedic surgery (e.g., total hip replacement), and chemical dependency treatment programs, are separated out from a managed care plan for procedure-specific or service-specific contracting. Specialty network providers are selected for their specialized expertise in that service or procedure, based on criteria and standards set by the payors. Specialty networks are usually very limited in size, and often are developed for high-cost care. Negotiated prices are usually tied to the procedure, with hospital, physician, ancillary services, and pharmacy bundled into one price (see *bundled billing*). Selected providers frequently share risk through a total capitated price, with cut-off levels ("stop-loss") for outliers.

Speech Pathologist

See also:
Speech Therapy

A specially trained health care professional who plans, directs, and conducts remedial programs designed to restore or improve the communication efficiency of patients with language and speech impairments arising from physiological or neurological disturbances and defective articulation. Licensure amd professional certification of clinical competence by the American Speech-Language and Hearing Association, requires academic training at the master's level, one year of field experience, and successful completion of a national examination.

Speech Therapy

See also:
Ancillary Service;
Speech Pathologist

The study, examination, and treatment of defects and diseases of the voice, speech, and spoken and written language, and the use of appropriate substitutional devices and treatment. Speech therapy is classified as a therapeutic *ancillary service*, like occupational and physicial therapy, by most managed care plans.

Staff Model HMO

See also:
Health Maintenance Organization (HMO)

A type of HMO that employs its own physicians to provide health care to enrollees. Generally, all ambulatory health services are provided under one roof, and all premiums and other revenues accrue to the HMO. Physician employees are compensated by salary and incentive programs.

Staff Privilege

See also:
Credentialing

The privilege granted by a hospital or other inpatient health care facility to a physician or other independent practitioner to join the facility's medical staff and admit private patients into the hospital. A practitioner is usually granted staff privileges after meeting certain standards, being accepted by the medical staff and the board of trustees, and agreeing to carry out certain duties for the hospital, such as teaching without pay or providing emergency or clinic services. Most community hospitals and other private hospitals are staffed by physicians in private practice who obtain access to hospital facilities in this manner. Often, a physician may have staff privileges at more than one hospital, and many hospitals have several different types of staff privileges, such as active, courtesy, associate, limited, etc.

S

Staffing Ratios/ Standards

See also:
Primary Care Physician / Practitioner (PCP)

An estimate of the number and types of *primary care providers* (PCP), including both physicians and non-physician practitioners, needed for a managed care plan. Often, staffing ratios or standards are expressed in terms of physician specialists needed for 1000 enrollees. For example, a large closed panel plan may use staffing ratios of 0.8 PCPs for 1,000 enrollees, whereas a smaller staff or group model HMO may have a staffing ratio of 1.3:1,000. The staffing ratio depends on a number of influencing factors, such as the size of the plan, availability of high quality PCPs, scope of clinical skills of PCPs in the panel, size of the Medicare population served. (Medicare members tend to utilize services more than non-Medicare members.)

Stakeholder

See also:
Provider;
Supplier;
Third Party Payor;
Vendor

Refers to any party either directly involved or having an interest (e.g., financial) in the health care delivery process. Though there are many different types of stakeholders, the majority can be classified into five main groups: 1) *providers* (e.g., hospitals, specialty providers, physicians); 2) *purchasers* (government agencies, employers); 3) *third party payors* (insurance carriers, managed care organizations); 4) *suppliers* (medical equipment and pharmaceutical manufacturers, distributors, and retailers, information systems *vendors*); and 5) *patients* (including the patient's family members). There also are other related stakeholders that do not fit well into any of these five categories. For example, brokers, managed care consultants, malpractice lawyers, politicians, and researchers may have a professional and/or financial interest in the health care delivery process, but cannot be classified as providers, purchasers, payors, suppliers, or patients.

Standard Benefits Package

See also:
Benefit(s) Package

A proposed uniform basic package of health benefits that would be guaranteed to all U.S. citizens. For example, the standard benefits package under consideration by the Clinton Administration would consist of a combination of medical services similar to a standard indemnity plan. This basic package would be the minimum standard level of services to which all Americans are entitled. In the event of a serious or catastrophic illness or injury, each family would pay an out-of-pocket amount which would be capped at a specified amount.

Standard Class Rate (SCR)

See also:
Premium;
Rating Process

The base revenue requirement for a group health plan on a per member or per employee basis. The SCR is factored into group demographic information to calculate monthly premiums.

Standard Industry Code (SIC)

A standardized classification code which the federal government developed to determine the type of industry of an employer group (e.g., retail, manufacturing, banking, health care, etc.). SIC codes are based on either products produced or operations performed.

Standard Insurance

See also:
Morbidity Tables;
Underwriting

Health insurance written on the basis of regular morbidity underwriting assumptions, using *morbidity tables* prepared by the Department of Health and Human Services (HHS), and issued at normal rates.

Standard Provision

Refers to certain provisions in health care contracts generally required by state statutes until superseded by a national uniform policy provision. (Contrast with *substandard risk.*)

Standard Risk

See also:
Substandard Risk;
Underwriting

Refers to a person who, according to an insurance company's underwriting standards, is entitled to insurance protection without extra premium rating or special restrictions.

Standards

See also:
Norms;
Peer Review Organization (PRO);
Performance Standards;
Pre-established Criteria .

Measures set by a competent authority as rules for determining quality, quantity or performance level. Conformity with standards is usually a condition of licensure, accreditation, or payment of services. In health care, standards may be defined in relation to the actual or predicted effects of care, performance or credentials of professional personnel, governance and administration of facilities and programs, etc. For example, in the *PRO* program, standards are professionally developed expressions of acceptable variation from *norms* or *pre-established criteria.*

State Disability Plan

A disability insurance plan for accident and sickness required by legislation in some states of those employers doing business in that particular state.

State Health Plan (SHP)

See also:
State Health Planning and Development Agency (SHPDA)

A comprehensive plan developed by a *state health planning and development agency (SHPDA),* which recommends a state's proposed strategic actions and expected changes in health resources over the next five years. The SHP also includes recommendations for implementing the strategies.

State Health Planning and Development Agency (SHPDA)

See also:
State Health Plan (SHP)

The state planning agency, organized under the National Health Planning and Resource Development Act, which prepares an annual *state health plan (SHP)* and state medical facilities plan. In some states, the SHPDA also performs *certificate of need (CON)* reviews.

State Insurance Department

The department of a state government responsible for regulating the insurance business in the state and providing public information on insurance.

Statewide Health Coordinating Board (SHCC)

See also:
State Health Planning and Development Agency (SHPDA)

A state advisory council of providers and consumers which supervises the work of the *state health planning and development agency (SHPDA)* and reviews and coordinates *state health plans (SHP)* and budgets.

Statistical Utilization Review (SUR)

See also:
Utilization Management (UM);
Utilization Review (UR)

A *utilization management* technique in which claims data are analyzed to determine which providers offer the most efficient and cost-effective patient care. SUR may include evaluation of physician office visit billing patterns by specialty to determine whether patterns agree with billing norms, review of return office visits generated by physicians by specialty, review of admission patterns of physicians who refer to specific hospitals, and evaluation of readmission rates for different hospitals. SUR may also include evaluation of utilization rates of pharmaceutical and diagnostic tests by condition at different hospitals.

Steerage

See also:
Benefit Differential;
Non-Participatory Provider (NonPar);
Steering Mechanisms

Refers to the differential amount between preferred and non-preferred benefits (i.e., *benefit differential)* designed to "steer" plan members to participating providers. For example, high steerage exists when plan members must share more of the cost of health services through higher deductibles or coinsurance when they elect to use *non-participatory providers.*

Steering Mechanisms

See also:
Benefit Differentials;
Steerage

Financial incentives for plan members to use preferred providers. Steering usually is accomplished through *benefit differentials* applied to the deductible, coinsurance, and coinsurance limits.

Step Therapy

In pharmacy, the process of treating a patient with the least expensive medication or therapy initially, then graduating to higher cost medications or therapies as required.

Step-Down Unit (SDU)

See also:
Skilled Nursing Facility (SNF)

A hospital ward or a section of a ward which is used as an alternative setting for patients requiring less care and monitoring than a patient who needs acute inpatient care. A step-down unit (SDU) operates in much the same way as a free-standing skilled nursing facility (SNF), but in many cases may offer greater convenience to the physician and the utilization review nurse by virtue of its location. Patients and family often find the SDU alternative more acceptable, too. The charge per day for the SDU usually is less than regular inpatient hospitalization because fewer resources are required.

Stop-Loss Reinsurance

See also:
Excess-of-Loss Reinsurance; Reinsurance

A type of *reinsurance* purchased by primary insurers to protect against excessive claims losses. Under this arrangement, reinsurance is written on an aggregate basis, and the reinsurer pays all or a percentage of the primary insurer's claims losses above a cumulative annual amount (e.g., above 110% or 125% of expected losses). The stop-loss may apply to an entire collection of risks, such as all primary insurance coverage in a state, or a self-insured employer's group health plan, or to any single component of a health plan. Stop-loss (aggregate) reinsurance is less common in insured health plans than *excess-of-loss reinsurance,* which is written on a per case basis. Many self-funded plans, however, being smaller than primary insurance companies, want protection against larger-than- expected losses on smaller claims, and often buy stop-loss reinsurance for their retained risk.

Subacute Care

See also:
Intermediate Care Facility (ICF);
International Subacute Healthcare Association (ISHA);
Skilled Nursing Facility (SNF)

An intermediate level of health care provided to medically fragile patients who are too ill to be cared for at home, but require medical and nursing services at a higher intensity level than is offered in a typical *skilled nursing facility (SNF).* Subacute care may be provided in long-term care hospitals, hospital-based skilled nursing units, transitional, or *intermediate care* units within community-based nursing facilities, and "swing" beds in hospitals eligible for the federal swing bed program. Subacute providers are regulated by state and federal requirements for either licensed hospital beds or skilled nursing beds. Two accrediting organizations are in the process of developing standards for subacute care, the *Joint Commission of Accreditation of Health Organizations (JCAHO)* and the Commission on Accreditation of Rehabilitation Facilities (CARF).

S

Subjective

Refers to characteristics that are based on professional judgments or opinions rather than empirically derived measures. For example, in outcomes research, patient satisfaction is a subjective measure of quality of care because it is based on patients' opinions and feelings rather than objective facts. (The antonym is *objective.*)

Subrogation

See also:
Coordination of Benefits (COB)

A legal right to recover from third parties the full amount or some proportion of benefits paid to an insured person. For example, if a plan member receives treatment through an HMO for injuries related to an automobile accident in which a third party was at fault, the HMO may file a claim with the negligent driver's automobile insurance company for the value of services provided to the injured plan member. Subrogation differs from *coordination of benefits (COB)* in that liability is shared under COB between parties on a contractual or legal basis, as opposed to subrogation which assigns the rights to another party.

Subscriber

See also:
Enrollee;
Member

The individual who is responsible for payment of premiums or whose employment is the basis for eligibility for membership in a group health plan. Sometimes called *member* or *enrollee.* However, not all members are subscribers, because the term "subscriber" does not refer to covered dependents who are members.

Subscriber Contract

See also:
Certificate of Coverage (COC)

A written agreement describing the covered person's health care policy. Also called a *subscriber certificate, member certificate*, or *certificate of coverage (COC).*

Substance Abuse

See also:
Mental Health / Substance Abuse (MH / SA)

The taking of alcohol or other intoxicants at dosages that place a person's social, economic, psychological and physical welfare in potential hazard, or endangers public health, morals, safety or welfare, or a combination of these.

Substandard Insurance

See also:
Standard Insurance

An individual health insurance policy issued with an extra premium or a special restriction to a person who does not qualify (i.e., does not meet the normal health requirements) for insurance at standard rates.

Substandard Risk

See also:
Standard Risk;
Substandard Insurance

Refers to an individual who, because of health history or physical limitations, does not measure up to the qualifications of a *standard risk,* which is someone who meets the normal health requirements of a standard health insurance policy.

Summary Plan Description (SPD)

See: **Explanation of Benefits (EOB)**

Superbill

See also:
Claim

A modified claim form that lists specific and/or specialty medical services provided by the physician. A superbill is not acceptable in place of the standard claim form required by managed care plans for reimbursement.

Supplemental Services

See also:
Surcharge

Optional services that a managed care plan may cover or provide in addition to its basic health services, which may involve additional charges, or *surcharges*.

Supplementary Medical Insurance Program (SMI)

See also:
Medicare

The voluntary part (Part B) of the *Medicare* program. SMI provides insurance benefits for physician and other medical services, such as home health care (up to 100 visits), outpatient hospital services, laboratory, pathology, and radiology services, and inpatient prescription drugs. SMI is financed from monthly premiums paid by enrollees and a matching amount from federal general revenues. During any calendar year, the program will pay 80% of the reasonable charges for all covered services after the insured pays a deductible. The name, *Part B*, derives from Part B of Title XVIII of the Social Security Act. Also called *Medicare Part B.*

Supplier

See also:
Vendor

An institution, individual, or agency that furnishes a medical item or service. In the Medicare program, suppliers are distinguished from providers (e.g., hospitals, skilled nursing facilities), and include independent laboratories, durable medical equipment and prosthesis providers, ambulance services, and providers of portable X-ray equipment. Suppliers are usually paid by insurance carriers and managed care plans on the basis of reasonable charges, rather than on a cost basis, as is often the case with providers.

Surcharge

See also:
Supplemental Services

An additional charge for optional or *supplemental services* provided over and above previously agreed upon charges for specified services.

Surgi-Center

See: **Free-Standing Outpatient Surgical Center**

Surgical Expense Insurance

See also:
Surgical Schedule

A type of health insurance which provides benefits toward the physician's or surgeon's operating fees. Benefits usually consist of specified amounts for each surgical procedure, as listed in the *surgical schedule.*

Surgical Schedule

See also:
Fee Schedule; Surgical Expense Insurance

A list of cash allowances attached to a *surgical expense insurance* policy, which are payable for various types of surgery. Typically, the maximum benefit amount is based on the severity of the surgical procedure. (Compare with *fee schedule.*)

Surplus

See also:
Risk Charge

The excess of an insurance company's assets (including any capital) over liabilities. Surpluses may be used for future dividends, business expansion, or to meet possible excessive losses. Surpluses may be developed intentionally by including an amount (*risk charge*) in the premium in excess of the standard premium needed to meet anticipated liabilities.

Swing-Out HMO

See: **Point-of-Service Plan (POS)**

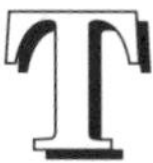

Table of Allowances

See also:
Fee Schedule; Scheduled Plan

A list of covered services developed by certain types of indemnity insurance plans (i.e., *scheduled plans*), whereby each health service is assigned a dollar amount representing the total obligation of the plan for payment for the service. In some cases, however, the assigned amount for a particular service may not represent the provider's full fee for that service.

Table Rates

See: **Age/Sex Rates (ASR)**

Target Group

See also:
Market Area

A defined population in a specified geographical area that is selected to receive special medical care based on perceived need or estimated demand for certain services.

Targeted Utilization Rates

See also:
Utilization

Rates set by managed care organizations that specify the number of admissions per 1,000 members, average length of stay (ALOS), hospital days per 1,000 members, use of ancillary services, and other measures of financial or utilization performance.

Tax Credit

See also:
Tax Deduction

A reduction of tax liability for federal income tax purposes. Several national health reform proposals include a tax credit which would allow individuals and businesses to reduce their taxes for certain medical expenses on a dollar-for-dollar basis. The effect of using a tax credit approach rather than a *tax deduction* method *is* that a tax credit provides individuals and businesses an equal benefit for each dollar spent on health care. Thus, a tax credit tends to favor lower incomes over higher, whereas a *tax deduction* has more value to a business or individual with a higher marginal tax rate. Also called *Medicredit*.

Tax Deduction

See also:
Tax Credit

A reduction in the income base upon which federal income tax is calculated. Health insurance expenditures are deductible by businesses as a business expense (currently 100% deductible for employers and 25% for self-employed individuals). Because the marginal tax rate is related to income and is greater for higher income individuals and businesses, the value of a tax deduction for medical care increases as income increases. Thus, the subsidy is effectively greater for the higher income person and the more profitable corporation.

Tax Equity and Fiscal Responsibility Act of 1982 (TEFRA)

See also:
Primary Payer

The federal law that created the current risk and cost provisions in HCFA's contracts with health plans. For example, TEFRA extended Medicare payment limits to ancillary services, added Medicare coverage of hospice care, and allowed Medicare to sign risk contracts with HMOs and competitive medical plans (CMPs). Another key TEFRA provision prohibits employers and health plans from requiring employees between the ages of 65 and 69 to use Medicare as the primary payer rather than the employer's group health plan.

Terminally Ill

See also:
Hospice Care

A medical prognosis of six months or less to live. Examples of terminal illnesses are: cancer, late stages of Alzheimer's Disease, and Lou Gehrig's Disease.

Termination Date

See also:
Effective Date

The date that a contract for a group health plan expires, as opposed to the *effective date*, which is the date that a health plan contract becomes in force. The term also may refer to the date that a member ceases to be eligible for coverage under the plan.

Tertiary Care

See also:
Primary Care;
Secondary Care

Highly specialized, complex, and technologically based medical services, e.g., heart, liver, or lung transplants, and other major surgical procedures, performed by highly specialized physicians in a hospital setting.

Therapeutic Equivalents

See also:
Chemical Equivalents

Drugs that contain different therapeutic modalities but provide the same pharmacological action or chemical effect when administered in similar therapeutic doses, as measured by the control of a symptom or illness. Sometimes called *chemical equivalents*, though not all therapeutic equivalents are *chemical equivalents* of their counterparts.

Therapeutic Substitution

See also:
Generic Substitution Program;
Therapeutic Equivalents

A managed care arrangement for drug benefits which allows the pharmacist to substitute a *therapeutic equivalent* (usually generic) for a drug prescribed by a physician but not on the managed care plan's drug formulary. The pharmacist must obtain the physician's permission prior to making the substitution.

Third Party Administrator (TPA)

See also:
Administrative Services Only Contract (ASO);
Third Party Payor

An independent firm which performs administrative services, such as premium collecting, claims processing, claims payment, membership services, utilization review, for employee health benefit plans and managed care plans. If claims payment is one of the services, the TPA is considered a *third party payor*. Unlike insurance carriers, TPAs do not underwrite the insurance risk. TPAs tend to be attractive to employers because their overhead is usually lower than commercial insurers. Also, they operate nationally with multiple offices offering localized services and usually are flexible in addressing client needs. Often, TPAs, particularly the large firms, are owned by another company (typically, insurers).

T

Third Party Payor

See also:
Payer (Payor)

Under a health benefit plan, a third party may be an insurance company, the government, a self-insured employer, or a managed care organization which is responsible for paying the costs of medical services provided to covered persons. The term derives from the fact that under normal market transactions, there usually are only two parties, the consumer (patient) and the supplier (provider); but in managed care contracting, a third party, such as a TPA, is also involved in the transaction and makes payments on behalf of the plan members.

Threshold for Action

See also:
Pre-established Criteria; Screening

In quality assessments or other patient care audits, the "threshold for action" is the minimum percentage of medical records that must meet *pre-established screening criteria* to indicate an acceptable clinical performance pattern. When actual performance does not equal or exceed the minimum percentage of records, the quality assurance review committee is obligated to take corrective action.

Time Limit

In claims processing, the period of time during which a notice of claim or proof of loss must be filed.

Title XIX

See also:
Medicaid; Medically Indigent

The section of the Social Security Act that describes the Medicaid program's coverage for eligible persons who may be *medically indigent.*

Title XVIII

See also:
Medicare

The section of the Social Security Act that describes the Medicare program's coverage for eligible persons (i.e., the aged, the blind, and the disabled).

Total Disability

See also:
Partial Disability

Disability due to injury, sickness or pregnancy which requires regular care and attendance of a participating physician, and renders the plan member, in the opinion of the participating physician, unable to perform the duties of his/her regular occupation, or engage in any other type of work. (Note: this wording may vary among insurance companies.)

Total Quality Management (TQM)

See also:
Continuous Quality Improvement (CQI); Quality Improvement Program (QIP)

A management philosophy and system for continuously improving performance at every level of every business process by focusing on meeting or exceeding customer expectations. Key elements of TQM include companywide *continuous quality improvement (CQI)* efforts (sometimes called a *quality improvement program*), self-directing work teams, employee involvement programs, flexible service delivery processes, quick changeover and adaptability, customer focus, supplier integration, and production cycle time reduction. Many health care organizations are implementing TQM programs as a competitive strategy.

Traditional Indemnity Insurance

See: **Fee-for-Service Insurance**

Transfer Agreement

A written arrangement between two institutions, such as a hospital and a nursing home, which facilitates the reciprocal transfer of patients from one institution to the other.

T

Transferability

A provision in some health insurance policies that gives the insured the right to receive from a new insurance contract the same benefits of the previous insurance policy when the subscriber has changed his/her place of residence.

Transitional Care Facility

See: **Intermediate Care Facility (ICF)**

Trauma

See also:
Emergency Care

A severe, life threatening injury which requires emergency care and possibly extensive lifesaving measures.

Treatment

The management and care of a patient for the purpose of combating disease or disorder.

Treatment Facility

See also:
Mental Health / Substance Abuse (MH / SA)

Refers to a residential or non-residential facility, or a licensed program authorized to provide treatment of mental illness or substance abuse in accordance with the legal jurisdiction where the treatment is received.

Trend Factor

See also:
Trending

Relates to the rate at which medical costs change due to certain influences, such as providers' prices (i.e., inflation), changes in the frequency and pattern of medical service utilization, cost-shifting, use of expensive medical technology, etc. A trend factor is applied as an annual adjustment factor to total incurred claims to represent the assumed or known change of these factors from one period to another.

Trending

See also:
Trend Factor

A type of calculation used by many managed care plans for predicting a group's future use of health services based on past use by applying a *trend factor*.

Triage

See also:
After-Hours Care; Triage Nurse

The process of assessing patients' conditions and classifying sick or injured persons according to severity and urgency of the condition in order to direct care and ensure the efficient use of medical and nursing staff and facilities. The term was originally used to describe a system used on the battlefront whereby casualties were sorted into groups of those who could wait for care, those who needed immediate care, and those who were beyond care. In the HMO context, triage refers to management of *after-hours care*, such as screening and referral, usually by telephone.

Triage Nurse

See also:
Triage

A nurse whose primary responsibility is screening patients to determine the type of care needed and the immediacy of the patient's need, in the professional opinion of the triage nurse.

Trim Points

See also:
Outliers

In DRGs, the minimum and maximum length of stay (LOS) for each DRG. Trim points are typically set at 5% of the total Medicare inpatient population that falls beyond the expected extremes of required hospitalization. Patients who fall outside of the trim points are considered *outliers*.

Triple Option Plan

See also:
Multiple Option Plan; Point-of-Service Plan (POS)

A type of managed care plan which allows members to choose any of three service options, HMO, PPO, or indemnity plan, each time they require medical care. Accountability for care is managed by a primary care physician. The scope of covered services is the same for each option. The only difference among options is the level of cost shared by the enrollee. An advantage of a triple option plan for employers is that it features a single set of benefits administered through a single carrier. Also called *point-of-service plan (POS)*.

Trust Fund

See also:
Multiple Employer Trust (MET)

A legal entity established to control, invest, and otherwise administer monies, securities, or other property for the benefit of others. The fund is operated under a trust agreement by trustees whose responsibility requires prudent administration of the fund's purpose. In group health, common trust funds are those created by unions and trade associations for the benefit of their members, and *multiple employer trusts (MET)* for the purpose of purchasing group health insurance for small employers. The Medicare program also is financed through trust funds. The Federal Hospital Insurance Fund finances Medicare Part A, and the Federal Supplementary Medical Insurance Trust Fund finances Medicare Part B.

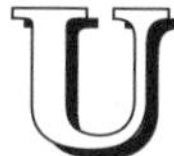

Ultrasound

See also:
Ancillary Services

A non-invasive diagnostic imaging technique which uses high frequency sound waves to "view" soft tissues of the body (mainly abdominal and pelvic areas), allowing physicians to see images in "real time," i.e., as they occur. Ultrasound is often used for fetal monitoring to monitor the fetus' heart beats, measure its gross size, and analyze its anatomical and functional characteristics.

Unallocated Benefit

See also:
Allocated Benefits; Ancillary Services

A provision in some insurance policies which allows reimbursement up to a maximum amount for the cost of all additional or extra miscellaneous hospital services (i.e., *ancillary services*) without specifying how much will be paid for each type of service. (Compare with *allocated benefits*.)

Unbundling

See also:
Bundled Billing

The practice by some providers of billing for multiple components of a medical service that normally are covered under one procedure code in order to increase revenues for the service. Generally, unbundling is considered an unethical practice. For example, a provider might bill additional charges for dressings and instruments which usually are included in the fee for a minor procedure while leaving the fee for the procedure itself unchanged.

Underinsured

See also:
Medically Indigent; Overinsurance

Describes the condition of individuals who have some health insurance coverage but, for a variety of reasons (high deductibles or copayments, restricted coverage, exclusions of certain conditions, caps on catastrophic benefits, etc.) have problems gaining access to health care. For example, a covered person may perceive that he/she cannot afford the deductible or copayment and, as a result, may forego needed treatment for an illness. A person is also underinsured when charges for catastrophic care exceed the cap on benefits included in his/her plan. Even though the underlying causes for underinsurance may be different (perceptual vs. actual), as in these two examples, the effects are the same–both have problems of access to health care.

Undertreatment

See also:
Overtreatment

Failure on the part of the provider to recommend and/or deliver at the proper time one or more of those services that, consistent with the diagnosis and treatment planning, are necessary and appropriate.

Underwriter

See also:
Underwriting

Usually refers to the company that receives premiums and accepts responsibility for the fulfillment of the health insurance policy contract. The term may also apply to an insurance company agent who sells the policy or an insurance company employee who has *underwriting* responsibility for determining whether or not the carrier should assume a particular risk.

Underwriting

See also:
Risk;
Underwriter

Refers to the process of identifying, evaluating and classifying the potential degree of risk represented by a group seeking insurance coverage, in order to determine appropriate pricing, risk assessment and administrative feasibility. The main purpose of underwriting is to assess the risks and make sure that the potential for loss is within the range for which the premiums were established. Underwriting can also refer to the acceptance of risk, as in the case of a policy that is underwritten by an insurance company.

Unearned Premium

See also:
Premium

The portion of a paid premium that applies to the unexpired portion of the policy term. Unearned premium also may refer to that portion of the paid premium for which benefits have not been received.

Uniform Bill / Patient Summary

See also:
Uniform Billing Code of 1992 (UB-92)

A medical services billing document which combines both patient billing information and medical data.

U

Uniform Billing Code of 1992 (UB-92)

See also:
Revenue Codes;
Uniform Bill / Patient Summary

A revised version of the *Uniform Billing Code of 1982 (UB-82),* which is the federal directive requiring hospitals to follow specific billing procedures and use a standard billing form, called the UB-92 form, for Medicare services. The new UB-92 form provides a summary of a claim and also a wide range of information regarding a particular admission to the provider facility. All billed services must be itemized on each form. The UB-92 form was implemented on October 1, 1993.

Uniform Hospital Discharge Data Set (UHDDS)

A defined set of data which provides a minimum description of a hospital episode of care or admission. Collection of UHDDS is required upon discharge for all hospital stays that are reimbursed under Medicare and Medicaid. The UHDDS includes data on age, sex, race, and residence of the patient, length of stay, diagnosis, responsible physicians, procedures performed, disposition of the patient, and sources of payment. The data are collected from the patient's medical record and abstracted in standard coded forms, called "discharge abstracts."

Uninsurable Risk

See also:
Insurable Risk

An individual or group that is not acceptable for insurance due to excessive risk. (Compare with *insurable risk*.)

Universal Access (UNAC)

See also:
Access;
American Health Security Act of 1993 (AHSA);
Cost-Shifting;
National Health Insurance

A component of most health care reform proposals which would extend health care coverage to all Americans, including the estimated 37 million or more who are either uninsured or underinsured. It is thought that universal access (UNAC) would eliminate the problem of *cost-shifting*, a practice that is prevalent among providers. Several alternatives for financing UNAC have been proposed, ranging from tax credits for employers, higher taxes on employers and employees, to a "single-payer" *national health insurance* program. For example, under the President Clinton's *American Health Security Act of 1993 (AHSA),* all U.S. citizens and legal residents would receive uninterrupted, comprehensive health coverage through state-established regional health alliances and corporate alliances, regardless of health or employment status. The coverage would be funded through contributions by individuals and families and by employers. The government would subsidize costs for many small and low-wage businesses and for individuals with incomes below 150% of the poverty line. Also known as *universal coverage.*

U

Universal Coverage

See: **American Health Security Act of 1993 (AHSA)** and **Universal Access (UNAC)**

Upcoding

See also:
DRG "Creep"

The unethical practice by some providers of billing for a procedure that has a greater reimbursement rate than the service actually performed, in order to increase revenues. Sometimes called *DRG "Creep."*

Urgent Care

See also:
After-Hours Care;
Emergency Care

Care for injury, illness, or another type of condition (usually not lifethreatening) which should be treated within 24 hours. Also refers to *after-hours care*, or to an HMO's classification of hospital admissions as urgent, semi-urgent, or elective.

Urgi-Center

See: **Free-Standing Emergency Medical Services Center** and **Urgent Care**

Usual, Customary, and Reasonable Fees (UCR)

See also:
Billed Charges;
Customary Charge;
Resource Based Relative Value Scale (RBRVS)

A reimbursement method used mostly in reference to fee-for-service reimbursement. A "usual" fee is one that an individual provider usually charges for a given service to a private patient. A fee is "customary" if it is in the range of usual fees charged by providers of similar training and experience in a geographical area. A fee is "reasonable" if it meets the two previous criteria or if, in the opinion of the medical or dental review committee, it is justifiable considering the special circumstances of the case in question. Most private health insurance plans use the UCR reimbursement approach, whereby they pay a physician's full charge if it does not exceed UCR charges. However, this is changing as more plans adopt the *RBRVS* method for physician reimbursement.

Utilization

See also:
Utilization Management (UM);
Utilization Rate;
Utilization Review (UR)

Refers to the use of health care services. Managed care plans typically regard utilization in terms of patterns or rates of use of a single service or type of service, such as hospital care, physician visits, or prescription drugs. Utilization may be expressed as the number of services used per year per 100 persons or per 1000 persons who are eligible for the services, or per eligible person. *Utilization rates* are established for health planning, budget review, and cost containment.

Utilization Management (UM)

See also:
Utilization;
Utilization Review (UR)

A management tool used by managed care plans involving the systematic process of reviewing and controlling patients' use of medical services and providers' use of medical resources. UM includes an array of techniques, such as second surgical opinion, preadmission certification, concurrent review, case management, discharge planning, and retrospective chart review. The term is used in preference to *utilization review (UR)* by managed care organizations to emphasize that patient care is not only reviewed, but processes are also managed in order to optimize efficiency and appropriateness of care.

Utilization Rate

See also:
Utilization

The volume of health care services used within a specific time period by a given population. Utilization rate is usually expressed as the number of units of service used per year per 1,000 persons eligible for the services. It also may be expressed as other types of ratios, for example, "per eligible person covered."

U

Utilization Review Accreditation Commission (URAC)

See also:
American Managed Care and Review Association (AMCRA);
Accreditation;
Utilization Review (UR);
Utilization Review Organization (URO)

An independent *accreditation* organization for *utilization review organizations (URO)*. URAC was established under the leadership of the *American Managed Care and Review Association (AMCRA)* as an alternative to state regulation and to introduce more consistency into *utilization review (UR)* processes. Its board of directors includes representatives from professional and trade associations of the major managed care stakeholders. URAC's goals are to encourage efficient and effective UR processes and provide a method of evaluation and accreditation for UR programs in order to improve the quality and efficiency of the interaction between the UR industry and health care providers, payors, and purchasers.
Address: URAC, 1130 Connecticut Ave., NW,
Suite 450, Washington, DC 20036
Phone: (202) 296-0120; Fax: (202) 296-0690

Utilization Review Organization (URO)

See also:
Utilization Review (UR)

An organization which conducts *utilization review (UR)* activites for managed care organizations. UROs determine certification of an admission, extension of stay in a medical facility, or provision of other health care services for a plan member. Physicians are usually employed by UROs on a part-time basis, often as consultants or advisors. Registered nurses (RNs) are heavily involved in first-level review decisions, but physicians become more involved during the second-level review and the appeals process. UROs frequently use commercially developed review criteria when making their recommendations.

Utilization Review (UR)

See also:
Utilization Management (UM); Prospective Review; Concurrent Review; Retrospective Review; Statistical Utilization Review (SUR)

A *utilization management (UM)* technique whereby trained health care professionals evaluate the appropriateness, quality, and medical necessity of services provided to plan members. Types of UR include: *prospective review*, in which a proposed schedule of treatment, including patient care, discharge plans, policies, or procedures that specify how care will be provided, is evaluated; *concurrent review,* in which routine medical procedures are monitored during the course of hospitalization or treatment to ensure that appropriate care is delivered; *retrospective review,* in which audits of selected medical records help payors assure that appropriate care was provided and billed; and *statistical utilization review (SUR),* in which claims data, like pricing and utilization, are analyzed to determine which providers offer the most efficient and cost-effective patient care.

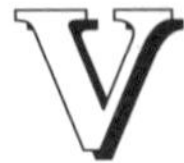

Validation Criteria

See also:
Combined Audit; Utilization Review (UR)

In utilization review, refers to health care standards that are stated in objective rather than descriptive terms in order to provide accurate evaluation. Validation criteria are used for determining whether a patient had the diagnosis or medical condition ascribed to him/her in the patient medical record.

Variance Report

See also:
Combined Audit; Validation Criteria

An audit committee report which lists medical record numbers that did or did not conform to *validation criteria*. Variation reports are accompanied by data retrieval comments as well as the audit committee's decisions about each record.

Variation

See also:
Screening; Variation Analysis

In utilization review, an instance in which information in a patient record does not conform to a screening criterion. The information in question may or may not be subsequently justified by an audit committee review.

Variation Analysis

See also:
Validation Criteria; Variation; Variation Record

An examination by the audit committee of certain patient medical records (referred to as *variation records*) which contain *variations* from *validation criteria* in order to determine which variations are clinically acceptable.

Variation Record

See also:
Validation Criteria

In utilization review, any patient medical record that reflects non-conformance to any *validation criterion*.

Vendor

See also:
Supplier

Any supplier or provider of health care services who is reimbursed directly by a third party payor for services rendered to eligible persons. A vendor may be an institution, agency, organization, or individual practitioner.

Vertical Integration

See also:
Continuum of Care; Horizontal Integration; Integrated Delivery System (IDS)

A provider strategy, usually accomplished through partnerships, joint ventures, and contractual arrangements, whereby providers establish a local or regional health care delivery network for the purpose of serving a geographically defined population. A vertically *integrated delivery system (IDS)* provides a *continuum of care,* that is, a full range of services and delivery settings to assist the patient in health, in sickness, and at death. By consolidating management functions and resources the IDS can achieve economies of scale and operate more cost-effectively. When used as a managed care strategy, vertical integration includes financing mechanisms as well as patient care services. It also requires either ownership of or alliances with a managed care plan or some other type of insurance contract (e.g., direct contracts with self-funded emloyers) which administers risk and captures market share to the IDS. (Compare with *horizontal integration.*)

V

Vision Care

See also:
Carve-Out Service

A type of group health plan which covers medical treatments relating to eye conditions. Most managed care plans accept opthalmologists (medical doctors) and optometrists and opticians (non-physicians) as qualified providers of vision care. Most plans limit eye examinations to not more than once in a 12 month period. New lenses and frames may be provided every 24 months. Often, vision care is provided by separately as a *carve-out service.*

Visiting Nurse Associations of America (VNAA)

See also:
Home Health Care;
Hospice Care

An umbrella organization for over 450 non-profit, community-based Visiting Nurse Associations (VNA) located nationwide in most urban and many rural areas. VNAs provide skilled nursing and other support services to patients of all ages, from infants to the elderly. Services include home health care, hospice care, infusion therapy, pediatric and maternal and child care programs, enterostomal therapy, and physical, speech, and occupational therapy. VNAs also provide personal care, homemaking, social services, and nutritional counseling. VNAA established a separate corporation, Visiting Nurse Preferred Care (VNPC), to serve as a contracting vehicle between local VNAs and third party payors. In addition, VNPC provides centralized intake, billing, case coordination, complaint resolution, and quality assurance.
Address: VNAA, 3801 E. Florida Ave., Suite 206, Denver, CO 80210
Phone: (303) 753-0218; Fax: (303) 753-0258

V

Volume Performance Standards (VPS)

See also:
Omnibus Budget Reconciliation Act (OBRA);
Performance Standards

Estimates of the annual rate of increase of Medicare expenditures for physician services, enacted as part of the *Omnibus Budget Reconciliation Act of 1989 (OBRA).* The purpose of VPS is to control the rate of increase in the volume and intensity of services provided to Medicare beneficiaries by providing a collective incentive for physicians to order fewer tests and procedures of limited value to patients.

Voluntary Enrollment

See also:
Dual Option;
Enrollment

Refers to an HMO enrollment process in which eligible persons willingly and explicitly choose to enroll in the HMO. Typically, employers offer an HMO as one of at least two group health plan options (i.e., *dual option* plan). Enrollment in the HMO must be completely voluntary for the employee.

Voluntary Hospital
See also:
Community Benefits

A not-for-profit hospital that is supported financially by voluntary gifts. Voluntary hospitals are exempt from many federal, state, and local taxes by virtue of their mission to provide *community benefits*. By contrast, for-profit hospitals are supported by investors for the purpose of gaining financial profits, and are taxed as corporations.

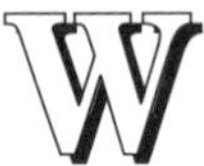

Waiting Period
See also:
Eligibility Date

A defined period of time that an individual must wait to become eligible for insurance coverage or to become eligible for a specific benefit after general coverage has commenced. For example, coverage under an employer's group health plan may not begin until an employee has been with the firm for more than thirty days. Another example is the two year waiting period required for disabled persons before they can be covered under Medicare. In this case, a person must be entitled to Social Security disability benefits for two years before medical benefits start. Also, some health insurance policies will not pay maternity benefits until nine months after the policy has been in force.

Waiver
See also:
Exclusions

An agreement attached to an insurance policy which exempts certain disabilities or injuries from coverage that normally are covered by the policy.

Waiver of Premium
See also:
Total Disability

A provision included in some health insurance policies which exempts the policyholder from paying premiums while the covered person is totally disabled during the life of the contract.

Washington Business Group on Health (WBGH)

A national non-profit health policy and research organization representing employers' interests in the formulation of health care policy. WBGH serves as a key source of information on corporate health care issues for Congress, the health care industry, academia, and the media. Membership consists of over 200 large employers representing all major industry segments. WBGH provides information on current health care initiatives and future trends to assist members in the purchase and provision of benefits to their employees. In addition, WBGH provides a forum through conferences, policy briefings, and symposia for the discussion of new health policy issues, cost management strategies, benefit design solutions, and health promotion ideas. WBGH also conducts research, identifies trends, collects and disseminates information, and provides long-range planning and analysis on many economic and social issues confronting employers.
Address: WBGH, 777 N. Capitol St., Suite 800, Wahington, DC 20002
Phone: (202) 408-9320; Fax: (202) 408-9332

W

Weighted Daily Census (WDC)

See also:
Average Daily Census (ADC)

The *average daily census (ADC)* weighted by the impact of outpatient volume.

Wellness

See also:
Health Promotion

A health care process which fosters awareness, influences attitudes, and identifies alternatives to unhealthy lifestyles so that individuals can make informed choices and change their behavior to achieve optimum physicial and mental health.

Wellness Program
See also:
Health Promotion;
Wellness

A broad range of employer-sponsored activities and facilities designed to promote safety and good health among employees. Wellness programs aim to increase worker morale and reduce the costs of accidents and ill health, such as absenteeism, lower productivity, and health care costs. *Wellness* and *health promotion* programs may include physical fitness programs and facilities, smoking cessation programs, health risk appraisals, diet information and weight loss programs, stress management, screenings for high blood pressure and cholesterol, etc.

Withhold

See: **Physician Contingency Reserve (PCR)**

Work-Up

Refers to a provider's assessment of a patient's condition, which typically includes history, physical findings, lab reports, and X-rays. The thoroughness and accuracy of the work-up is stressed by HMOs, especially when a patient is being referred to an out-of-network provider. The work-up by the HMO accompanies the referral, and sometimes also determines whether the referral receives authorization by the managed care plan.

Workers' Compensation (WC)

See also:
Occupational Diseases

A state-governed insurance program designed to address work-related injuries. Under the workers' compensation (WC) system, employers assume the cost of medical treatment and wage losses arising from injuries and diseases related to a worker's employment, regardless of who is at fault. In return, employees give up the right to sue their employer, even if injuries are a result of employer negligence. WC programs are financed by the employers that are covered under the plans. WC programs are mandatory under most states' law. In recent years, the medical costs of WC have risen faster than health care costs in general. As a result, more employers are turning to managed care techniques to contain their escalating WC costs. Several national health reform plans, including the American Health Security Act of 1993, encourage treatment of work-related injuries through HMOs and other managed care networks. Support also is growing among many employers and legislators to integrate the WC system into the mainstream health care system so that medical coverage for occupational injuries would be provided by health insurers rather than WC insurers. WC insurers, however, would still provide wage replacement benefits.

W

Wraparound Coverage

See also:
Fee-for-Service Insurance (FFS)

A type of *fee-for-service insurance* coverage to supplement benefits offered by a group or staff model HMO, or other basic health plan, such as Blue Cross/Blue Shield or Medicare. Wraparound coverage provides plan members limited coverage for services provided by non-participatory providers.

Written Premiums

Refers to the entire amount of premiums due in a given year for all health care policies issued by an insurance company.

Z

Zero Balanced Reimbursement Account (ZEBRA)

See also:
Cafeteria Plan;
Flexible Benefit Plan (Flex Plan);
Section 125 Plan;
Self-Funded Plan

A type of *flexible benefit plan* provided by employers who self-insure and pay for care as it is given. ZEBRAs permit employees to receive spending account reimbursements. Typical ZEBRA features include: delaying salary reductions until expenses are submitted, eliminating forfeiture of unused spending accounts, and an unlimited ceiling for benefits. Unlike a *cafeteria plan*, a ZEBRA is not a tax-qualified plan structured under *Section 125* of the Internal Revenue Code. Funds spent for an employee under a ZEBRA plan are taxable to the employee, and the employer is liable for withholding income tax on benefits.

Section 2
Acronyms & Abbreviations

Commonly used acronyms and abbreviations are listed alphabetically and spelled out in this section. When only the acronym is familiar to the user, the user should refer to this section first to find the formal name, then turn to that term in **Part I, Section 2—Terms** for a full explanation.

AAFP American Association of Family Physicians

AAPCC Adjusted Average Per Capital Cost

AAPHO American Association of Physician-Hospital Organizations

AAPI American Accreditation Program, Inc.

AAPPO American Association of Preferred Provider Organizations

ACR Adjusted Community Rating

ADA Americans with Disabilities Act

ADC Average Daily Census

ADL Activities of Daily Living

ADS Alternative Delivery Systems

AFHHA American Federation of Home Health Agencies

AHA American Hospital Association

AHCA American Health Care Association

AHCPR Agency for Health Care Policy and Research

AHP Accountable Health Partnership *or* Plan

AHSA American Health Security Act of 1993

ALOS Average Length of Stay

AMA American Medical Association

AMCP Academy of Managed Care Pharmacy

AMCRA American Managed Care and Review Association

AMPRA American Medical Peer Review Association

ANA American Nurses Association

AOB Assignment of Benefits

APG Ambulatory Patient Group

APN Advanced Practice Nurse

APR Average Payment Rate

ASHRM American Society for Healthcare Risk Management

ASO Administrative Services Only Contract

ASR Age/Sex Rates

AWP Average Wholesale Price

BC/BS Blue Cross/Blue Shield Association *or* Plan

CABG Coronary Artery Bypass Graft Project

CAM Catchment Area Management Project

CAP Capitation

CAT Computerized Axial Tomography

CCN Community Care Network

CCP Coordinated Care Program

CCRC Continuing Care Retirement Community Program

CCU Coronary Care Unit

CHAM-PUS Civilian Health and Medical Program of the Uniformed Services

CHC Community Health Center

CHMIS Community Health Managed Information System

CM Case Management

CM Case Manager

CMP Competitive Medical Plan

CMSA Case Management Society of America

CNM Certified Nurse Midwife

Co-Pay Copayment

COA Certificate of Authority

COB Coordination of Benefits

COBRA Consolidated Omnibus Budget Reconciliation Act of 1985

COC Certificate of Coverage

COI Certificate of Insurance

CON Certificate of Need

COPC Community Oriented Primary Care Program

CPI Consumer Price Index

CPI-MCS Consumer Price Index-Medical Care Services

CPR Customary, Prevailing, and Reasonable

CPT-4 Physician's Current Procedural Terminology, 4th Edition

CQI Continuous Quality Improvement

CRC Community Rating by Class

CRI CHAMPUS Reform Initiative

CSR Continued Stay Review

CTD Cumulative Trauma Disorder

CWW Clinic Without Walls

D.C. Doctor of Chiropractic

D.O. Doctor of Osteopathy

DAW Dispense As Written

DC Dual Choice

DCI Duplicate Coverage Inquiry

DME Durable Medical Equipment

DMO Dental Maintenance Organization

DOS Date of Service

DPR Drug Price Review

DRG Diagnosis-Related Group

DUM Drug Utilization Management

DUR Drug Utilization Review

EAP Employee Assistance Program

EAPA Employee Assistance Professionals Association, Inc.

EASNA Employee Assistance Society of North America

EBIS Employee Benefits Information System

EBR Employee Benefits Representative

EBRI Employee Benefits Research Institute

ECF Extended Care Facility

EDI Electronic Data Interchange

EMO Exclusive Multiple Option

EMS Emergency Medical Services

EOB Explanation of Benefits

EofI Evidence of Insurability

EPO Exclusive Provider Organization

EPSDT Early and Periodic Screening, Diagnosis, and Treatment

ERISA Employee Retirement Income Security Act

ESRD End Stage Renal Disease

FAHS Federation of American Health Systems

FAS-106 Financial Accounting Standards - Rule 106

Fee Max Fee Maximum

FEHBP Federal Employee Health Benefits Program

FFS Fee-for-Service Reimbursement

FI Fiscal Intermediary

FMC Foundation for Medical Care

FP Family Practice

FPP Faculty Practice Plan

FQHMO Federally Qualified HMO

FTE Full Time Equivalent

GDP Gross Domestic Product

GHAA Group Health Association of America

GNP Gross National Product

GP General Practitioner

GPCI Geographic Practice Cost Index

GPWW Group Practice Without Walls

HCCP Health Care Prepayment Plan

HCFA Health Care Financing Administration

HCP Health Care Plan

HCPCS HCFA Common Procedural Coding System

HCQI Health Care Quality Improvement Act of 1986

HEDIS Health Plan Employer Data & Information Set

HHA Home Healthcare Agency

HHS Health & Human Services Department

HI Horizontal Integration

HIAA Health Insurance Association of America

HIN Health Insurance Network

HIO Health Insuring Organization

HIPC Health Insurance Purchasing Cooperative

HISB Health Insurance Standards Board

HMO Health Maintenance Organization

HOI Health Outcomes Institute

HPA Hospital-Physician Alliance

HPNS Healthcare Provider Networks Section of the AHA

HRSA Health Resources and Services Administration

HSA Health Services Agreement

HSB Health Standards Board

IAF Industry Adjustment Factor

IBNR Incurred But Not Reported

ICD-9 International Classification of Disease, 9th Edition

ICF Intermediate Care Facility

ICMA Individual Case Management Association

ICU Intensive Care Unit

IDS Integrated Delivery System

IFEBP International Foundation of Employee Benefit Plans

IP Inpatient

IPA Independent Practice Association

ISHA International Subacute Healthcare Association

JCAHO Joint Commission on Accreditation of Healthcare Organizations

JPA Joint Powers Authority

LCAH Life Care at Home Program

LCM Large Case Management

LOB Line of Business

LOS Length of Stay

LPN Licensed Practical Nurse

LTC Long-Term Care

LVN Licensed Vocational Nurse

MA Medical Assistant

MAC Maximum Allowable Cost

MAP Maximum Allowable Payment

MaxLOS Maximum Length of Stay

MCE Medical Care Evaluation

MCM Medical Case Management

MCO Managed Care Organization

MCP Managed Care Plan

MDC Major Diagnostic Categories

MERP Medical Expense Reimbursement Plan

MET Multiple Employer Trust

MEWA Multiple Employer Welfare Association

MGMA Medical Group Management Association

MH/SA Mental Health/ Substance Abuse

MHCA Managed Health Care Association

MHSS Military Health Services System

MIC Maternal & Infant Care

MIG Medicare-Insured Group

MIP Managed Indemnity Plan

MIS Management Information System

MLP Mid-Level Practitioner

MLR Medical Loss Ratio

MM Member Months

MOB	Maintenance of Benefits Plan
MOR	Monthly Operating Report
MPP	Minimum Premium Plan
MRI	Magnetic Resonance Imaging
MSA	Metropolitan Statistical Area
MSO	Management Service Organization
NAEBA	National Association of Employee Benefit Administrators
NAHC	National Association for Home Care
NAIC	National Association of Insurance Commissioners
NAMCP	National Association of Managed Care Physicians
NBCFH	National Business Coalition Forum on Health
NCI	Nursing Care Institution
NCPA	National Center for Policy Analysis
NCQA	National Committee for Quality Assurance
NDC	National Drug Code
NHB	National Health Board
NHLA	National Health Lawyers Association
NLR	Net Loss Ratio
NMHCC	National Managed Health Care Congress
NonPar	Non-Participatory Provider
NP	Nurse Practitioner
NPDB	National Practitioner Data Bank
OBRA	Omnibus Reconciliation Act
OHMO	Office of Health Maintenance Organizations
OMSB	Outcomes Management Standards Board
OOA	Out-of-Area Services
OON	Out-of-Network Services

OOP Out-of-Pocket Payments

OP Outpatient

OPHCOO Office of Prepaid Health Care

OPL Other Party Liability

OPM Office of Personnel Management

OSC Organized System of Care

OSCR On-Site Concurrent Review

OSHA Occupational Safety and Health Act

OT Occupational Therapist

OTC Over-the-Counter Drug

P&T Pharmacy & Therapeutic Committee

PA Physician's Assistant

PAS Professional Activities Survey

PAS Preadmission Screening Program

PAT Preadmission Testing

PCLR Paid Claims Loss Ratio

PCN Primary Care Network

PCP Primary Care Physician/ Practitioner

PCPM Per Contract Per Month

PCR Physician Contingency Reserve

PET Positron Emission Tomography

PHCO Physician-Hospital-Community Organization

PHO Physician-Hospital Organization

PLI Professional Liability Insurance

PMA Pharmaceutical Manufacturers Association

PMPM Per Member Per Month

POP Premium-Only Plan

POS Point-of-Service Plan

PPI-H Producer Price Index-Hospital

PPO Preferred Provider Organization

PPS Prospective Payment System

PRO Peer Review Organization

ProPAC Prospective Payment Assessment Commission

PSAO Pharmacy Services Administration Organization

PSRO Professional Standards Review Organization

PTMPY Per Thousand Members Per Year

QA Quality Assurance

QIP Quality Improvement Program

QMB Qualified Medicare Beneficiary

QRC Quality Review Committee

R&C Reasonable & Customary Charge

RAP Radiologists, Anaesthesiologists, and Pathologists

RBRVS Resource Based Relative Value Scale

RCF Residential Care Facility

Retro Retrospective Rate Derivation

RFI Request for Information

RFP Request for Proposal

RIMS Risk and Insurance Management Society

RN Registered Nurse

RVS Relative Value of Services

RWJF Robert Wood Johnson Foundation

SAP Service Assessment Program

SCR Standard Class Rate

SDU Step-Down Unit

SHP State Health Plan

SHPDA State Health Planning & Development Agency

SHPM Society for Healthcare Planning &Marketing

SIC Standard Industry Code

SIIA Self-Insurance Institute of America

SIW Service Intensity Weights

SMI Supplementary Medical Insurance Program

SNF Skilled Nursing Facility

SOBRA Sixth Omnibus Reconciliation Act

SPBA Society of Professional Benefit Administrators

SSO Second Surgical Opinion

SSSG Similarly-Sized Subscriber Group

SUR Statistical Utilization Review

TEFRA Tax Equity & Fiscal Responsibility Act of 1982

TPA Third Party Administrator

TQM Total Quality Management

UB-92 Uniform Billing Code of 1992

UCR Usual, Customary, and Reasonable Fees

UHDDS Uniform Hospital Discharge Data Set

UM Utilization Management

UNAC Universal Access

UR Utilization Review

URAC Utilization Review Accreditation Commission

URO Utilization Review Organization

VNAA Visiting Nurse Association of America

VPS Volume Performance Standards

WBGH Washington Business Group on Health

WDC Weighted Daily Census

ZEBRA Zero Balanced Reimbursement Account

Section 1
Trade Associations

Organizations representing various managed care stakeholders and their interests are listed alphabetically in this section. The organizations can also be found in both the **Terms** and the **Acronyms** sections (1 and 2) in **Part I.**

Academy of Managed Care Pharmacy (AMCP)

A national professional society of pharmacists, organized for the purpose of promoting the development and advancement of pharmaceutical care in managed health care environments. The AMCP had 1700 members in 1993, representing approximately 200 managed care organizations. AMCP provides educational programs, including two annual national conferences and several regional conferences, bimonthly newsletters, and other resources useful to members. AMCP also monitors legislative issues that impact managed care pharmacy and is proactive in the development of position statements and related resource materials.

Address: AMCP, 1321 Duke Street, Suite 305, Alexandria, VA 22314
Phone: (703) 683-8416 or (800) TAP-AMCP
Fax: (703) 683-8417

American Association of Physician-Hospital Organizations (AAPHO)

See also:
Physician-Hospital Organization (PHO)

A recently established (in 1993) national organization which serves as a resource for networking, education and advocacy for physicians, hospitals, and *Physician-Hospital Organizations (PHO)* interested in furthering the development of PHOs. Creation of the AAPHO was spearheaded by executives at the Piedmont Healthcare Organization, a PHO affiliated with Piedmont Hospital in Atlanta, GA. Its first symposium has been scheduled for February 10-11, 1994, in Atlanta, GA. Additional educational conferences are planned throughout the year. AAPHO publications include a quarterly newsletter (AAPHO Insights), a membership directory, and a consultants directory. The AAPHO also offers members preferred rates for consultants.

Address: AAPHO, P. O. Box 4913, Glen Allen, VA 23058-4913
Phone: (800) 722-0376; Fax: (804) 747-5316

American Association of Preferred Provider Organizations (AAPPO)

See also:
Preferred Provider Organization (PPO)

A national trade organization representing *preferred provider organizations (PPO)* and their partners in managed care. Members include PPOs, insurance companies, physicians, hospitals, consultants, TPAs, and pharmaceutical companies. The AAPPO's mission is to provide direction and assistance to and for the managed healthcare industry through education, information, research, and advocacy. Membership benefits include: national conferences, regional seminars, publications (e.g., Directory of Operational PPOs), research activities, and networking opportunities. The AAPPO represents its members' views to the trade and media, monitors the legislative and regulatory environment, and advocates PPOs and related issues at national, state, and local levels.
Address: AAPPO, 1101 Connecticut Ave., Suite 700, Washington, DC 20036
Phone: (202) 429-5133; Fax: (202) 429-5108

American Federation of Home Health Agencies (AFHHA)

See also:
Home Healthcare Agency (HHA);
Visiting Nurse Association of America (VNAA)

A national trade organization representing the interests of Medicare-certified *home healthcare agencies (HHA)* in legislative and regulatory processes. Membership includes a variety of home health providers, including free-standing, hospital-based, and chain HHAs, *visiting nurse association (VNA)* agencies, and county agencies. Membership also is open to state home health associations, vendors, consultants, and individuals. Its primary objective is to influence public policy processes. AFHHA monitors national legislative developments, provides technical advice and support, educational seminars, and networking opportunities to members. Publications include the Insider newsletter, and legislative and regulatory "alerts."
Address: AFHHA, 1320 Fenwick Lane, Suite 100, Silver Spring, MD 20910
Phone: (301) 588-1454; Fax: (301) 588-4732

American Health Care Association (AHCA)

See also:
Long-Term Care (LTC)

A national federation of 51 associations (in 1993) representing 11,000 non-profit and for-profit *long- term care (LTC)* providers. AHCA promotes standards for LTC professionals and quality care for LTC residents. AHCA provides members information on legislative and regulatory policy and initiatives, health care management, facility administration, and pertinent products and services through its monthly publication, Provider, and biweekly newsletter, AHCA Notes. AHCA also publishes career training and educational materials relating to LTC.
Address: AHCA, 1201 L Street, NW,
Washington, DC 20005-4014
Phone: (202) 842-4444; Fax: (202) 842-3860

American Hospital Association (AHA)

A national trade association representing nearly 5,500 hospitals, including general and specialized hospitals, corporate health care systems, and hospital-related providers of preacute and postacute services. AHA also has 16 personal membership groups and various associate memberships. The AHA represents members interests with legislators and government agencies, the media, and accrediting organizations (e.g., JCAHO) and develops policy positions and research. AHA publications, such as Hospitals & Health Networks, address current issues facing hospitals. Educational activities include national conferences, satellite teleconferences, and a resource center containing a collection of health care administration literature.
Address: AHA, 840 N. Lake Shore Drive,
Chicago, IL 60611
Phone: (312) 280-6000; Fax: (312) 280-3061

American Managed Care and Review Association (AMCRA)

A national trade organization representing approximately 500 managed care organizations (in 1993), including HMOs, PPOs, IPAs, UROs, HIOs, FMCs, and PROs. Membership also includes allied health professionals who provide services to the managed care industry. AMCRA provides educational programs, conducts research, promotes utilization review and quality assurance, communicates with legislative and governmental agencies, and serves as an information clearinghouse on legislative issues, industry trends, and statistics.
Address: AMCRA, 1227 25th St., NW, Suite 610, Washington, DC 20037
Phone: (202) 728-0506; Fax: (202) 728-0609

American Medical Association (AMA)

See also:
Doctor of Osteopathy (D.O.);
Physician

The nation's largest professional organization for *physicians*, representing approximately 42% of the nation's 615,000 physicians in 1993. Membership is open to doctors of medicine (M.D.) and *doctors of osteopathy (D.O.)*. The AMA offers opportunities for education, professional development, and political advocacy. The AMA's proposal for health care reform calls for universal access to health care, malpractice reform, and controlled spending through market forces rather than mandatory caps on physicians' fees.
Address: AMA, 515 N. State Street, Chicago, IL 60610
Phone: (312) 464-5000; Fax: (312) 464-5837

American Medical Peer Review Association (AMPRA)

See also:
Peer Review Organization (PRO)

A national trade association representing federally designated *peer review organizations (PRO)* under contract with the Medicare program. AMPRA's stated goal is to insure the incorporation of quality of care evaluation in national health care reform. AMPRA serves as the national policy voice for PROs, physician-directed medical review organizations, and individuals supportive of quality evaluation and improvement in peer review activities. The association works closely with various government agencies in developing regulations, budgets, and policies governing medical review programs in the public sector. Membership services include an information clearinghouse, educational seminars, national conferences, research on quality assessment tools and technology, and informational publications.
Address: AMPRA, 810 First St., NE, Suite 410, Wahington, DC 20002
Phone: (202) 371-5610; Fax: (202) 371-8954

American Nurses Association (ANA)

See also:
Registered Nurse (RN)

A professional organization representing *registered nurses (RN)* through its 53 constituent associations, called State Nurses Associations (SNA). Through its SNAs, the ANA offers group purchasing advantages, develops nursing policy, lobbies for nursing and health care issues at the state and national levels, and presses for equitable salaries and working conditions. ANA also provides networking opportunities, research and educational events, legislative updates, publications, and certification programs through the American Nurses Credentialing Center (ANCC).
Address: ANA, 600 Maryland Ave., SW, Suite 100W, Washington, DC 20024-2571
Phone: (800) 274-4464; Fax: (202) 554-2262

American Society for Healthcare Risk Management (ASHRM)

See also:
American Hospital Association (AHA); Risk Management

A national professional society, organized as a component of the *American Hospital Association (AHA)*, representing professionals and students who are actively involved or otherwise interested in health care *risk management*. Members are hospital and other health care risk managers, nursing executives, administrators, commercial underwriters, insurance brokers, legal counsel, and consultants. The ASHRM provides its members a forum for the exchange of ideas and proven methodologies in health care risk management. Educational programs include annual conferences, workshops, seminars, research, publications, and other resources. ASHRM also monitors legislation affecting health care risk management and insurance.
Address: ASHRM, 840 N. Lake Shore Drive, Chicago, IL 60611
Phone: (312) 280-6430; Fax: (312) 280-4151

Case Management Society of America (CMSA)

See also:
Case Manager (CM)

A professional society for *case managers (CM)* employed by managed care organizations, insurers, and case management companies and in independent practice. Membership benefits include educational and networking opportunities through annual conferences and educational forums. CMSA also represents members' interests in government affairs and legislative issues, and offers a Certification for Case Managers (CCM) credentialing program.
Address: CMSA, 1101 17th St., NW, Suite 1200, Washington, DC 20036
Phone: (202) 296-9200; Fax: (202) 296-0023

Employee Assistance Professionals Association, Inc. (EAPA)

See also:
Employee Assistance Program (EAP)

A trade association representing the professional interests of practitioners in the *employee assistance program (EAP)* field. EAPA provides its members (7,000 in 1993) networking and educational opportunities, develops training programs for EAP staff, publishes literature to promote a better understanding of EAPs, and serves as an information resource on EAPs.
Address: EAPA, Inc., 4601 N. Fairfax Dr., Suite 1001, Arlington, VA 22203
Phone: (703) 522-6272; Fax: (703) 522-4585

Employee Assistance Society of North America (EASNA)

See also:
Employee Assistance Program (EAP)

A professional organization for *Employee Assistance Program (EAP)* practitioners. EASNA offers its members educational and professional development programs, networking opportunities, and legislative advocacy. The organization has developed a set of EAP standards and offers an EAP accreditation program to purchasers and clients of EAPs in order to promote excellence in EAP programming.
Address: EASNA, 2728 Phillips, Berkley, MI 48072
Phone: (313) 545-3888; Fax: (n/a by request)

Federation of American Health Systems (FAHS)

A trade association representing the investor-owned hospital and health care systems industry, consisting of more than 1,400 institutions in all 50 states, the District of Columbia, Puerto Rico, and 11 foreign nations. The primary function of the FAHS is to advocate members' interests to Congress, the Executive Branch, the media, academia, and the public. The FAHS also serves as a clearinghouse for vital information on health care issues and industry positions, policies, and statistics. FAHS conducts research on various health issues, prepares position papers and other informational literature, and offers educational opportunities through an Annual Conference and Business Exposition and through its publications, including the bimonthly Health Systems Review, biweeekly Hotline newsletter of Washington events, monthly newsletter, State-to-State, reporting on legislative and regulatory events. FAHS supports market-based health care reform through managed competition instead of global budgets or price controls.

Address: FAHS, 1111 19th Street, NW, Suite 402, Washington DC 20036
Phone: (202) 833-3090; Fax: (202) 861-0063

Group Health Association of America, Inc. (GHAA)

A trade association representing the interests of HMOs in policy and legislative issues affecting the managed care industry. GHAA had 350 HMO members in 1993. In addition to HMO organizational membership, GHAA offers individual, student, international, corporate supporting memberships, and memberships for state managed care associations. GHAA provides legislative representation at federal and state levels, legal counsel, educational programs, research, and publications. The organization also maintains a library of managed care resources, which is open to members and non-members. GHAA publications include the annual National Directory of HMOs and HMO Industry Profile, a bimonthly HMO Magazine, and a biweekly *HMO Managers Letter*.
Address: GHAA, 1129 20th St., NW, Suite 600, Washington, DC 20036
Phone: (202) 778-3200; Fax: (202) 331-7487

Health Insurance Association of America (HIAA)

A national trade association for commercial health insurers. HIAA serves as a forum for public policy development, represents members' views to Congress, state legislatures, and the public, and influences legislation and regulations. HIAA also conducts research, publishes literature and policy analyses on health insurance trends, and advises members about pertinent government activities and public opinion on health care issues. A managed care advocacy network was developed in 1991 to cultivate the managed care environment. A Managed Care Resource Center serves as a clearinghouse for publications and materials on managed care. Other membership services include: networking opportunities, educational seminars, workshops, publications (e.g., Source Book of Health Insurance Data), on-line database information services, and a consumer helpline.
Address: HIAA, 1025 Connecticut Ave., NW, Washington, DC 20036-3998
Phone: (202) 223-7800; Fax: (202) 223-7897

Healthcare Provider Networks Section of the AHA (HPNS)

See also:
Society for Healthcare Planning and Marketing (SHPM)

A special membership subgroup of the American Hospital Association's *Society for Healthcare Planning and Marketing (SHPM)*, formed in 1992 for health care professionals dealing with managed care issues. HPNS addresses policies and critical issues of managed care. HPNS also serves as an information clearinghouse on managed care services and activities, and encourages the exchange of information vital to the successful advancement of managed care programs.
Address: HPNS, 840 N. Lake Shore Drive, Chicago, IL 60611
Phone: (312) 280-6086; Fax: (312) 280-6252

HMO Group, The

See also:
Federally Qualified HMO;
Health Plan Employer Data & Information Set (HEDIS)

A national alliance of 21 non-profit, federally qualified, independent group and staff model HMOs, formed in 1984 for the purpose of defining and strengthening the HMOs' quality and performance. The HMO Group offers members on-site reviews to assure delivery of quality care and service, customer satisfaction surveys, a central resource for information sharing on operational and product concerns, publications, educational conferences, and seminars. The HMO Group participated in the development of the *Health Plan Employer Data and Information Set (HEDIS),* a standardized data collection and reporting system for assuring purchasers of the quality of HMO services.
Address: The HMO Group, 100 Albany St., Suite 230, New Brunswick, NJ 08901
Phone: (908) 220-1388; Fax: (908) 220-0298

Individual Case Management Association (ICMA)

See also:
Case Manager (CM)

A professional organization which represents independently practicing *case managers (CM)* who contract with managed care organizations, self-funded employers, and insurers to provide CM services in a specific geographical area. ICMA offers members educational programs, including seminars and a national conference, a national databank of CMs and other medical and disability management professionals, networking opportunities, publications (CM Trends, The Case Manager, ICMA Directory), and other personal training and resource materials. ICMA initiated a national CM certification program in 1991, which now is administered by the Certified Insurance Rehabilitation Specialists Commission.
Address: ICMA, 10809 Executive Center Drive
Suite 105, Little Rock, AR 72211-6020
Phone: (501) 227-5553; Fax: (501) 227-8362

International Foundation of Employee Benefit Plans (IFEBP)

An educational association in the employee benefits field which offers its members information services, publications, educational programs, on-line benefits database, research publications, certification program, and a student "I.F. Interns" program. Total membership in 1993 consisted of 34,000 individuals representing more than 7,500 trust funds, public employee funds, corporations, and professional firms throughout the U.S. and Canada.
Address: IFEBP, 18700 W. Bluemound Road, P.O. Box 69, Brookfield, WI 53008-0069
Phone: (414) 786-6700; Fax: (414) 786-2990

International Subacute Healthcare Association (ISHA)

See also:
Intermediate Care Facility (ICF); Subacute Care

A trade association representing the interests of subacute and transitional providers and practitioners. ISHA is developing industry standards and guidelines to help payors, health care personnel, and the public identify quality subacute and transitional care providers. Membership services include: educational seminars and materials, networking opportunities, a resource library, monthly newsletter, and legislative and regulatory representation regarding policies that impact subacute and transitional care providers.
Address: ISHA, 4040 W. 70th Street, Minneapolis, MN 55435
Phone: (612) 926-1773; Fax: (612) 926-1624

Managed Health Care Association (MHCA)

See also:
Health Plan Employer Data and Information Set (HEDIS); Outcomes Management System (OMS)

A national trade organization representing over 120 large employers which have implemented or are considering managed care programs. MHCA provides a forum for exchange of ideas and experiences on how to manage health care programs for better results, with an emphasis on measuring quality, service levels, cost performance, and employee and patient satisfaction. MHCA fosters education and training for benefits and health care management professionals through annual national meetings, dissemination of information on public policy and innovative managed care projects, and publications. MHCA also is involved in projects for standardizing outcomes and managed care data measures, such as the *Outcomes Management System (OMS)* project and the *Health Plan Employer Data and Information Set (HEDIS)* for measuring the value of managed care to employers.
Address: MHCA, 1225 Eye St., NW, Suite 300, Washington DC 20005
Phone: (202) 371-8232; Fax: (202) 842-0621

Medical Group Management Association (MGMA)

See also:
Group Practice

A trade organization representing physicians, administrators, CEOs, office managers and other professionals involved in medical *group practices*. MGMA provides its members networking, professional development, and educational opportunities through special interest Assemblies, Alliances, and Societies, (e.g., the American College of Medical Group Administrators), and through seminars and an annual national conference. A Library Resource Center provides information on relevant legislative and regulatory activities, and consulting assistance in identifying and solving management problems. Technical support and advice for improving health care delivery and administrative processes of members' group practices is offered though its Center for Research in Ambulatory Care Administration. MGMA publishes the bimonthly MGM Journal, a monthly newspaper (MGM Update), a membership directory, and other subscription publications.
Address: MGMA, 104 Inverness Terrace East, Englewood, CO 80112-5306
Phone: (303) 799-1111; Fax: (303) 643-4427

National Association for Home Care (NAHC)

See also:
Home Healthcare Agency (HHA);
Hospice Care

A national trade association for providers of home health and hospice care services. Associate memberships are open to businesses, corporations, and others that supply products or services to home care and hospice providers. NAHC offers educational and networking oportunities through an annual meeting, ten regional conferences, and an annual legislative and regulatory conference and computer exposition. Its publications include a weekly and biweekly newsletters, monthly Caring Magazine and Homecare News, and health care reform updates.
Address: NAHC, 519 C Street, NE,
Washington, DC 20002-5809
Phone: (202) 547-7424; Fax: (202) 547-3540

National Association of Employee Benefit Administrators (NAEBA)

See also:
COBRA;
Third Party Administrator (TPA)

A trade association of independent *third party administrator* firms that specialize in design, administration, and reporting of self-funded group health plans, utilization management, and managed care programs. NAEBA offers members advisory assistance in *COBRA* and other regulatory matters, provides educational services, e.g., employee benefits communication program, and access to a nationwide network of PPOs. Member firms subscribe to common standards of practice and utilize a common technology for claims processing.
Address: NAEBA, 12416 S. Harlem Avenue,
Palos Heights, IL 60463
Phone: (708) 448-8077; Fax: (708) 448-8158

National Association of Insurance Commissioners (NAIC)

See also:
Model HMO Act

A trade organization of state insurance regulators which provides a forum for developing national uniformity in the regulation of insurance. NAIC develops model laws, regulations, and guidelines for insurance companies, prepaid managed care plans, and state legislatures. For example, NAIC adopted the *Model HMO Act* in 1972, which authorizes the establishment of HMOs and provides for an ongoing regulatory monitoring system. NAIC also adopted a PPO Arrangements Model Act, which has regulatory requirements applicable to PPO-type products underwritten or administered by insurance companies. NAIC also monitors federal activity which affects insurance regulation, maintains market-based information systems, produces consumer guides, conducts research, provides educational programs, performs solvency surveillance and financial regulation, and offers an accreditation program.
Address: NAIC, 120 W. 12th St., Suite 1100,
Kansas City, MO 64105
Phone: (816) 842-3600; Fax: (816) 471-7004

National Association of Managed Care Physicians (NAMCP)

A professional organization representing physicians who practice in a managed care environment. NAMCP provides a forum for managed care physicians to communicate concerns about the changing health care environment, facilitates physicians' integration into managed care delivery systems, and fosters continuous improvement in the quality of care through research, communication, and education. Members include physicians, medical directors, health care professionals employed by or contracting with managed care plans, and employers interested in managed care.
Address: NAMCP, Innsbrook Corporate Center,
5040 Sadler Rd., Suite 103, Glen Allen, VA 23060-6124
Phone: (804) 527-1905; Fax: (804) 747-5316

National Business Coalition Forum on Health (NBCFH)

See also:
Business Coalition

A national organization representing over 70 non-profit *business coalitions* nationwide with a mission of community-based health care reform. NBCFH supports federal and state reform initiatives, consumer education and responsibility, universal coverage funded through tax credits and tax deductions, and improved measurement systems that enable health care purchasers to compare performance of providers. The organization promotes community-based health reform to employers in cities where business coalitions have not yet emerged, involves providers in the collection and analysis of information on quality, costs, and improvement of the community's health, ensures that health benefit plans contain consumer incentives to use high-value providers, and informs policymakers of the importance of community-based health care reform.
Address: NBCFH, 1015 18th Street, NW, Suite 450, Washington, DC 20036
Phone: (202) 775-9300; Fax: (202) 775-1569

National Health Lawyers Association (NHLA)

A national professional association for attorneys who are interested in or who practice health care law. The NHLA offers members educational, networking, and advocacy opportunities. NHLA also publishes newsletters, texts, references, and other educational materials covering many areas of health law as it relates to managed care. NHLA publications are suitable for the health law "expert" and the "novice."
Address: NHLA, 1620 Eye Street, NW, Suite 900, Washington, DC 20006
Phone: (202) 833-1100; Fax: (202) 833-1105

Pharmaceutical Manufacturers Association (PMA)

A national trade association representing the interests of more than 100 research-based pharmaceutical companies. PMA supports public policies that foster private research and development, free trade principles, and full protection of intellectual property rights. PMA studies the medical, social, and economic benefits provided by specific drugs and by the pharmaceutical industry in general, and communicates this information to policy-makers and the public. PMA favors a managed competition approach to health care reform, inclusion of prescription drug benefits in the standard benefit package, and voluntary efforts by drug companies rather than government price controls and global budgets to restrain price increases.
Address: PMA, 100 15th Street, NW,
Washington, DC 20005
Phone: (202) 835-3400; Fax: (202) 785-4834

Risk and Insurance Management Society, Inc. (RIMS)

A professional association for employee benefits managers of large corporations, non-profit and public sector institutions, and government agencies. RIMS offers educational courses, conferences and seminars, monitors regulatory and legislative developments, and represents members' positions concerning reform issues that affect the stability of the risk management and 770
employee benefits environment. RIMS also conducts research on emerging trends and publishes periodicals, books, and other resources. RIMS' Associate in Risk Management Program professional credentialing program is offered in conjunction with the Insurance Institute of America.
Address: RIMS, 205 East 42nd St., 15th Floor,
New York, NY 10017
Phone: (212) 286-9292; Fax: (212) 986-9716

Self-Insurance Institute of America, Inc. (SIIA)

See also:
Self-Funded Plan

A national trade association for the three principal entities of the self-insurance industry–employers, third party administrators (TPA), and reinsurance companies. SIIA's goal is to improve the quality and efficiency of *self-funded plans* and enhance public acceptance of this viable alternative to conventional insurance. SIAA activities include: educational and training programs, publications, and representation of members' concerns in federal legislative and regulatory areas through a political action program.
Address: SIIA, P.O. Box 15466, Santa Ana, CA 92705
Phone: (714) 261-2553; Fax: (714) 261-2594

Society for Health-care Planning and Marketing (SHPM)

See also:
American Hospital Association (AHA); Healthcare Provider Networks Section (HPNS)

A professional membership group of the *American Hospital Association (AHA)* serving the needs of health care planning and marketing executives. SHPM offers educational programs on strategic planning, marketing, physician services, sales, and managed care. It also provides access to the AHA's information resources and serves as an information clearinghouse. A newly formed (in 1992) subgroup, the *Healthcare Provider Networks Section (HPNS),* serves the professional interests of managed care executives. SHPM sponsors an annual Managed Care Forum to meet the educational needs of HPNS members.
Address: SHPM, 840 N. Lake Shore Drive
Chicago, IL 60611
Phone: (312) 280-6086; Fax: (312) 280-6252

Society of Professional Benefit Administrators (SPBA)

See also:
Third Party Administrator (TPA)

A national association of about 450 independent *third party administrator* (TPA) firms that manage clients' employee benefit plans. Members' clients include small businesses, large corporations, unions, and association-sponsored plans in every industry and profession. SPBA provides leadership in cost-containment efforts, cost-efficient administration techniques for pension and health benefit plans, as well as understanding of complex government compliance requirements.
Address: SPBA, Two Wisconsin Circle, Suite 670, Chevy Chase, MD 20815
Phone: (301) 718-7722; Fax: (301) 718-9440

Visiting Nurse Associations of America (VNAA)

See also:
Home Health Care; Hospice Care

An umbrella organization for over 450 non-profit, community-based Visiting Nurse Associations (VNA) located nationwide in most urban and many rural areas. VNAs provide skilled nursing and other support services to patients of all ages, from infants to the elderly. Services include home health care, hospice care, infusion therapy, pediatric and maternal and child care programs, enterostomal therapy, and physical, speech, and occupational therapy. VNAs also provide personal care, homemaking, social services, and nutritional counseling. VNAA established a separate corporation, Visiting Nurse Preferred Care (VNPC), to serve as a contracting vehicle between local VNAs and third party payors. In addition, VNPC provides centralized intake, billing, case coordination, complaint resolution, and quality assurance.
Address: VNAA, 3801 E. Florida Ave., Suite 206, Denver, CO 80210
Phone: (303) 753-0218; Fax: (303) 753-0258

Section 2
Policy & Research Organizations

Organizations involved in managed care policy research and policy-making are listed alphabetically in this section. Each of these organizations is also listed by name in **Part I, Section 1—Terms,** and by acronym (if applicable) in **Part I, Section 2—Acronyms & Abbreviations.**

Alpha Center

See also:
Robert Wood Johnson Foundation (RWJF)

A private, non-profit health policy organization, which sponsors demonstration and research programs, facilitates changes in health care financing and organization, provides technical assistance and guidance on health policy issues, and disseminates policy and research results through briefings and publications targeted to national audiences. Alpha Center directs the "Health Care for the Uninsured Program" and the "Changes in Health Care Financing and Organization" initiatives for the *Robert Wood Johnson Foundation (RWJF).* The organization also conducts educational conferences and workshops on health policy and planning topics, provides a resource center and library for information on a wide variety of health-related topics, and distributes a newsletter, Health Care for the Uninsured Program Update.
Address: Alpha Center, 1350 Connecticut Ave., NW, Suite 1100, Washington, DC 20036
Phone: (202) 296-1818; Fax: (202) 296-1825

Employee Benefits Research Institute (EBRI)

A non-profit, non-partisan public policy research organization which provides educational and research materials about employee benefits to employers, employees, retired workers, public officials, members of the press, academics, and the general public. Through books, policy forums, and a monthly subscription service, EBRI contributes to the formulation of effective and responsible employer-sponsored health, welfare, and retirement policies.
Address: EBRI, 2121 K Street, NW, Suite 600 Washington, DC 20037-1896
Phone: (202) 659-0670; Fax: (202) 775-6312

Health Outcomes Institute (HOI)

See also:
InterStudy;
Outcomes Management System (OMS);
Outcomes Measurement;
Outcomes Research

A privately funded health policy think tank, organized in February, 1993, which specializes in *outcomes research.* HOI is continuing to develop and distribute the *Outcomes Management System (OMS)* methodology for measuring outcomes, which originally was developed by *InterStudy*, a health care research organization. The OMS measures patient function, well-being, and clinical status. OMS methodology relies on quality-of-life self-assessments by patients who complete a questionnaire and condition-specific clinical forms completed by physicians.
Address: HOI, 2001 Killebrew Dr., Suite 122, Bloomington, MN 55425
Phone: (612) 858-9188; Fax: (612) 858-9189

InterStudy

See also:
Health Outcomes Institute (HOI);
Jackson Hole Group (JHG);
Outcomes Management System (OMS);
Outcomes Research

A research organization specializing in managed care research, particularly of HMOs. InterStudy maintains a database on HMO enrollment, characteristics, and qualification status. Its publications include the Competitive Edge, an HMO directory, and a series of monographs on outcomes research. InterStudy developed a methodology for measuring health care outcomes, called the *Outcomes Management System (OMS),* which was turned over to *Health Outcomes Institute*, an *outcomes research* organization, in February, 1993. In July, 1993, InterStudy was acquired by Decision Resources, a health care publishing and consulting firm in Waltham, MA.
Address: InterStudy, 2901 Metro Drive, Suite 400, Bloomington, MN 55331
Phone: (612) 858-9291; Fax: (612) 854-5698

National Managed Health Care Congress (NMHCC)

A national educational forum which focuses on the entire managed health care industry and its various constituents (e.g., employers, hospitals, physicians, managed care organizations pharmacists, military, MIS vendors). NMHCC seeks to provide common ground in the search for mutually successful solutions among managed care stakeholders. NMHCC holds a national conference in Washington DC in spring and several regional conferences throughout the year.
Address: NMHCC, 1000 Winter Street, Suite 4000, Waltham, MA 02154
Phone: (617) 487-6700; Fax: (617) 487-6709

Robert Wood Johnson Foundation (RWJF)

A national health philanthropy which designs, funds, and evaluates health services and health policy research projects which support the organization's four main goals: 1) improving access for Americans of all ages to basic health care; 2) improving service systems for people with chronic health conditions; 3) promoting health and preventing disease by reducing harm caused by substance abuse; and 4) addressing the problem of rising health care costs. The RWJF publishes a quarterly newsletter, Advances, sponsors educational forums, and offers educational materials produced by RWJF-funded projects to the public.
Address: RWJF, College Road, P.O. Box 2316, Princeton, NJ 08543-2316
Phone: (609) 452-8701

Washington Business Group on Health (WBGH)

A national non-profit health policy and research organization representing employers' interests in the formulation of health care policy. WBGH serves as a key source of information on corporate health care issues for Congress, the health care industry, academia, and the media. Membership consists of over 200 large employers representing all major industry segments. WBGH provides information on current health care initiatives and future trends to assist members in the purchase and provision of benefits to their employees. In addition, WBGH provides a forum through conferences, policy briefings, and symposia for the discussion of new health policy issues, cost management strategies, benefit design solutions, and health promotion ideas. WBGH also conducts research, identifies trends, collects and disseminates information, and provides long-range planning and analysis on many economic and social issues confronting employers.
Address: WBGH, 777 N. Capitol St., Suite 800, Wahington, DC 20002
Phone: (202) 408-9320; Fax: (202) 408-9332

Section 3
Accrediting Organizations

Organizations and agencies that provide accreditation for managed care organizations are listed alphabetically in this section and also in the **Terms** and **Acronyms** sections in the first part of this book (**Part I, Sections 1 and 2**).

American Accreditation Program, Inc. (AAPI)

See also:
Accreditation;
American Association of Preferred Provider Organizations (AAPPO)

A corporation which offers an *accreditation* program for PPOs seeking an endorsement of their products in the marketplace. The AAPI was created by the *American Association of Preferred Provider Organizations (AAPPO)* in 1989 in response to criticism of PPOs by health care purchasers and industry competitors. Unlike HMOs, PPOs are not federally regulated, and state-level regulation varies considerably. AAPI has developed a set of eight criteria, or *standards*, that define a managed care PPO: 1) network; 2) legal structure; 3) provider selection; 4) utilization management; 5) administration capabilities; 6) financial solvency; 7) quality assessment; and 8) payment methodologies. Medicare and some large employers both have used AAPI's protocols as a basis for selecting and contracting with PPOs. "Pure discount" PPO networks are not considered "managed care" by the AAPI, and therefore, are not eligible for its accreditation program.
Address: AAPI, 2270 Cedar Cove Court,
Reston, VA 22091
Phone: (703) 860-5900; Fax: (703) 860-5901

Joint Commission on Accreditation of Healthcare Organizations (JCAHO)

See also:
Accreditation;
Integrated Delivery System (IDS)

A private, non-profit organization which functions as the main accrediting body for hospitals and other provider facilities. JCAHO's seeks to improve health care quality by publishing national standards, surveying facilities on request, and awarding accreditation to those that demonstrate compliance with the standards. JCAHO accreditation is voluntary, but is a required for participation in Medicare. JCAHO is now developing accreditation standards applicable specifically to health care networks, which are being published in 1994. Relevant performance measures will be developed, tested, and introduced over the next two years.
Address: JCAHO, One Renaissance Blvd.,
Oakbrook Terrace, IL 60181
Phone: (708) 916-5800; Fax: (708) 916-5644

National Committee for Quality Assurance (NCQA)

See also:
Accreditation;
Health Plan Employer Data and Information Set (HEDIS)

An independent, non-profit HMO accrediting organization, composed of independent health care quality experts, employers, labor union officials, and consumer representatives. NCQA's *accreditation* program is designed for most HMO models. Its accreditation standards focus on: 1) quality improvement; 2) credentialing; 3) members' rights and responsibilities; 4) utilization management; 5) preventive health services; 6) medical records. NCQA uses a standardized data reporting system, the *Health Plan Employer Data and Information Set (HEDIS),* to measure HMO quality.
Address: NCQA, 1350 New York Ave., Suite 700,
Washington, DC 20005
Phone: (202) 628-5788; Fax: (202) 628-0344

Utilization Review Accreditation Commission (URAC)

See also:
American Managed Care and Review Association (AMCRA); Accreditation; Utilization Review (UR); Utilization Review Organization (URO)

An independent *accreditation* organization for *utilization review organizations (URO).* URAC was established under the leadership of the *American Managed Care and Review Association (AMCRA)* as an alternative to state regulation and to introduce more consistency into *utilization review (UR)* processes. Its board of directors includes representatives from professional and trade associations of the major managed care stakeholders. URAC's goals are to encourage efficient and effective UR processes and provide a method of evaluation and accreditation for UR programs in order to improve the quality and efficiency of the interaction between the UR industry and health care providers, payors, and purchasers.
Address: URAC, 1130 Connecticut Ave., NW,
Suite 450, Washington, DC 20036
Phone: (202) 296-0120; Fax: (202) 296-0690

Section 4
Government Agencies

Government agencies that are involved with managed care legislation or administration are listed alphabetically in this section. The agencies may also be found in both the **Terms** and the **Acronyms** sections in **Part I, Sections 1 and 2.**

Agency for Health Care Policy and Research (AHCPR)

An agency of the U. S. Public Health Service within the Department of Health & Human Services (HHS), which funds and conducts health services research and assessments of health care technologies. ACHPR programs focus on: 1) development, publication, and dissemination of clinical practice guidelines and information for patients (in English and Spanish); 2) medical treatment effectiveness studies, including 14 Patient Outcomes Research Teams (PORTs), which assess alternative methods for diagnosing, treating, managing, or preventing a particular condition; 3) evaluation of risks, benefits, and effectiveness of new or unestablished medical devices, procedures, and other health care technologies; 4) programs that address access to health services, cost, financing, and quality of care. The agency offers numerous publications through its AHCPR Publications Clearinghouse that describe its programs and present research findings and technology assessments.
Address: AHCPR, 2101 E. Jefferson St., Suite 501, Rockville, MD 20852
Phone: (800) 358-9295; Fax: (301) 594-2283

Health and Human Services Department (HHS)

See also:
Health Care Financing Administration (HCFA); Office of Prepaid Health Care Operations & Oversight (OPHCOO)

A federal Cabinet level agency which oversees government health care programs and activities, including Social Security, Medicare, and Medicaid. The *Health Care Financing Administration (HCFA), Health Resources & Services Administration (HRSA),* and *Office of Prepaid Health Care Operations & Oversight (OPHCOO)* (formerly known as the *Office of Health Maintenance Organizations)* are part of the HHS, which once was named the Health, Education and Welfare Department (HEW).
Address: HHS, 200 Independence Ave., SW, Washington, DC 20201
Phone: (202) 619-0257; Fax: *(by department)*

Health Care Financing Administration (HCFA)

See also:
Health and Human Services Department (HHS);
Medicaid;
Medicare

The federal agency responsible for administering *Medicare* and overseeing states' administration of *Medicaid*. HCFA also manages HMO qualification, the Utilization and Quality Control Peer Review, and a variety of other health care financing and quality assurance programs. HCFA is a part of the *Health and Human Services Department (HHS)*. HCFA's main office is in Washington, DC. The agency also has a Research Office and an Office of Statistics & Data Management, both located in Baltimore, Maryland.
Main office phone: (202) 727-0735
Research Office phone: (410) 966-6674
Office of Statistics & Data Mgmt. phone: (410) 597-3855

Health Resources and Services Administration (HRSA)

See also:
Maternal and Infant Care Program (MIC);
National Practitioner Data Bank (NPDB)

A federal agency of the U.S. Public Health Service within the Department of Health and Human Services (HHS) responsible for developing primary health care services and resources, protecting and improving the health of mothers, infants, and children, improving access to care for the medically underserved and those with special needs, and maintaining a high quality of health care nationally. The HRSA has five major operating components: Office of the Administrator; Bureau of Health Professions, which administers the *National Practitioner Data Bank (NPDB)*; Bureau of Health Resources Development; Bureau of Primary Health Care; Maternal & Child Health Bureau.
Address: HRSA, 5600 Fishers Lane, Room 14-45, Parklawn Bldg., Rockville, MD 20857
Phone: (301) 443-2086; Fax: (301) 443-1989

National Practitioner Data Bank (NPDB)

See also:
Health Care Quality Improvement Act of 1986 (HCQI);
Health Resources and Services Administration (HRSA)

A repository for certain information related to the professional competence and conduct of physicians, dentists, and other health care practitioners. The NPDB was established by the *Health Care Quality Improvement Act of 1986 (HCQI)* to serve as a background reference for health care organizations to check practice records of physicians and practitioners being considered for employment. The HCQI Act requires hospitals, health plans, malpractice insurers, state licensing boards, and professional societies to report malpractice claims settlements, licensure sanctions, and restrictions against practice privileges of a practitioner. NPDB information is confidential, and access is restricted to certain eligible entities. NPDB is administered by the *Health Resources and Services Administration (HRSA),* a federal agency in the Department of Health and Human Services.
Address: NPDB, P.O. Box 6050, Camarillo, CA 93011
Phone: (800) 767-6732

Office of Health Maintenance Organizations (OHMO)

See also:
Office of Prepaid Health Care Operations and Oversight (OPHCOO)

The former name for the federal agency within the U.S. Department of Health and Human Services which oversees federal activity relating to HMOs. OHMO has been reorganized, initially as the *Office of Prepaid Health Care (OPHC),* and now as the *Office of Prepaid Health Care Operations and Oversight (OPHCOO).*

Office of Personnel Management (OPM)

See also:
Federal Employees Health Benefit Program (FEHBP); Similarly-Sized Subscriber Group (SSSG)

The federal agency authorized to offer certain choices of health benefits plans to federal employees. (See *Federal Employees Health Benefit Program*) OPM can offer both experience-rated plans and comprehensive community-rated plans (mostly HMOs). OPM does not engage in a competitive bidding process. Instead, it relies on rates set by other managed care contractors and compares OPM rates with other HMO groups of similar size and benefits. HMOs participating in FEHBP are subject to periodic audit by the OPM, which involves reviews of state and federal rate filings, actual billings to commercial accounts, and rate worksheets used in developing the HMO's premium.

Office of Prepaid Health Care Operations and Oversight (OPHCOO)

See also:
Office of Health Maintenance Organizations (OHMO)

A division of the HCFA which is responsible for overseeing federal HMO qualification, CMP eligibility, ongoing HMO and CMP regulation, and employer compliance efforts. OPHCOO also administers Medicare Risk contracts, determines the capitation formula and reimbursement policies, and oversees the operation of the prepaid health information system. HMO qualification and CMP eligibility review processes are complex and can take six months to a year, or longer. Review areas include: legal, financial viability, health services delivery, and marketing. The OPHCOO was once a part of the U.S. Public Health Service, and called the *Office of Health Maintenance Organizations (OHMO).*
Address: OPHCOO, Cohen Building, Room 4406,
330 Independence Ave., SW, Washington, DC 20201
Phone: (202) 619-0845; Fax: (202) 619-2011

Peer Review Organization (PRO)

See also:
Peer Review;
Professional Standards Review Organization (PRSO);
Tax Equity and Fiscal Responsibility Act of 1982 (TEFRA)

A federal program established by the *Tax Equity and Fiscal Responsibility Act of 1982 (TEFRA),* which monitors the medical necessity and quality of services provided to Medicare and Medicaid beneficiaries under the prospective payment reimbursement system. PROs also validate provider coding assignments that affect Medicare reimbursement. In 1984, HCFA began contracting with peer review organizations (PRO) in every state. Hospitals are required to contract with a PRO in its state as a condition of receiving Medicare payments. PRO reviews evaluate care provided by hospitals, hospital outpatient departments, ambulatory surgical centers, emergency rooms, skilled nursing facilities, home health agencies, risk-sharing HMOs and competitive medical plans. Along with utilization and quality reviews, PROs are also responsible for investigating complaints by Medicare beneficiaries regarding the quality of care provided by HMOs. PROs are held responsible for maintaining and lowering admission rates, reducing lengths of stay, and ensuring against inadequate treatment.

Professional Standards Review Organization (PSRO)

See also:
Peer Review Organization (PRO);
Tax Equity and Fiscal Responsibility Act of 1982 (TEFRA)

A government-mandated organization (now defunct) composed of local practicing physicians. PSROs contracted with HCFA to review health care services covered under Medicare, Medicaid, and Maternal and Infant Care (MIC) programs. The goal was to confirm that services paid for under these programs was medically necessary, appropriate, and consistent with professionally recognized standards of quality. The federal requirement for establishing PSROs was added to the Social Security Act in 1972. The program was repealed by the *Tax Equity and Fiscal Responsibility Act of 1982 (TEFRA)* and PSROs were replaced by *Peer Review Organizations (PRO).*

Prospective Payment Assessment Commission (ProPAC)

See also:
Medicare;
Prospective Payment System (PPS)

A government agency established under the Social Security Act Amendments of 1983 to advise Congress and the Department of Health and Human Services regarding maintaining and updating *Medicare* payments to hospitals and other provider facilities. Because ProPAC is an appointed advisory body, it has no regulatory or appeals authority. ProPAC's responsibilities include Medicare inpatient and outpatient hospital payment policies, prospective payment policies for skilled nursing facilities and home health services, and payment for services furnished in end stage renal disease (ESRD) facilities. ProPAC also is required to examine uncompensated care and Medicaid payments, and their relationship to the financial condition of hospitals.

Address: ProPAC, 300 7th Street, SW, Suite 301-B, Washington, DC 20024
Phone: (202) 401-8986; Fax: (202) 401-8739

Add terms to the *Managed Care Desk Reference*

The ***Managed Care Desk Reference*** defines and describes terms used by managed care "stakeholders" from many different businesses, professions, and specialties and lists many of the key organizations currently involved in some capacity in the managed health care.

We have tried to be as inclusive as possible, but, given the rapid changes in our health care system, we know that we must have missed some terms or organizations that you think should be in this book.

Please help us improve the next edition by sending us the terms or names of organizations which you believe should be included. It would be helpful if you would also tell us how these terms are used and how the organizations are involved in managed health care.

Mail or fax your suggestions or any comments about the definitions to:

HCS Publications
P.O. Box 781982
Dallas, TX 75378-1982
Fax: (214) 747-8123

Your feedback is important to us. We appreciate your assistance!

Ordering Information

Are there others in your company who should be using the ***Managed Care Desk Reference***? Use the coupon on the right to order additional copies of the ***Managed Care Desk Reference*** at $65 per book. Be sure to include your payment plus shipping charge. Your book(s) will be sent to you as soon as we receive your payment.

Order by Mail:
Mail the completed coupon with your payment to: **HCS Publications**
P.O. Box 781982
Dallas, TX 75378-1982

Order by Phone or Fax:
For faster service, call (214) 748-9408 or fax your order to (214) 747-8123. Be sure to have your VISA or MasterCard account number ready, since all orders must be prepaid.

Shipping Charges:
Please add $4.00 to the purchase price for the first book and $1.00 for each additional book.

Sales Tax:
Texas residents add 8%, or your local rate to the purchase price.

Delivery:
In most cases, books will be shipped by UPS ground service. Please allow 1-2 weeks for delivery. We will be glad to ship your books overnight or second day delivery for an additional charge. Large quantities will be shipped via the fastest and most economical ground method, at the purchaser's expense. Please allow additional time for delivery.

Discounts:
Quantity discounts are also available. To see if your order qualifies for a discount, call our Customer Service Department at (214) 748-9408, between 9:00 a.m. and 5:00 p.m. CST, Monday through Friday.

Return Policy:
You may receive a full credit or refund only if you return your books to us in unmarked, good condition (suitable for resale) within 15 days. Please enclose a copy of your invoice plus a note explaining why you are returning the books. Shipping charges are not refundable.

Missing Order Coupons:
If the order coupon is missing from this book, please call (214) 748-9408. We will gladly send you additional coupons or take your order by phone.

For a faster response, you may FAX a copy of this form to 214/747-8123

Risk-Free* Order Coupon

☑ **Yes!** Please send me _____ copies of the ***Managed Care Desk Reference*** at $65 per book.

My Name: ____________________

Title: ____________________

Company: ____________________

Address: ____________________

____

City, State Zip: ____________________

Phone: ____________________

My preferred payment method:

☐ Check ☐ Visa ☐ MasterCard Expiration Date: ____ / ____ (MO. / YR.)

Card Number: ☐☐☐☐☐☐☐☐☐☐☐☐☐☐☐☐

____
Cardholder's name as it appears on the card

✗ ____________________
Signature of cardholder (required for credit card purchase)

Payment Worksheet

	Quantity		Amount
Managed Care Desk Reference	_____	x $65.00 =	$ _______
Texas Residents, Add Sales Tax of 8%			$ _______
Shipping & Handling:			
First Copy:			$ 4.00
Additional Copies:	_____	x $1.00 =	$ _______
Overnight Charge:	Add $15.00		$ _______
Total Amount:			$ _______

*** Money-Back Guarantee: You may return your book(s) within 15 days in saleable condition and receive a prompt refund if you are not satisfied.**

To help us serve you better, please indicate the "managed care stakeholder" category that best describes your job function or your organization:

- ☐ A. Clinic/Hospital
- ☐ B. Individual Physician
- ☐ C. Physician Group Practice
- ☐ D. HMO/PPO
- ☐ E. Utilization Review Co.
- ☐ F. Commercial Employer
- ☐ G. Business Coalition
- ☐ H. Human Resources
- ☐ I. Employee Benefits Manager
- ☐ J. Risk Management
- ☐ K. Network Management
- ☐ L. Third Party Administration
- ☐ M. Trade or Professional Assn.
- ☐ N. Consulting Service
- ☐ O. Labor Union Official
- ☐ P. Attorney/Legal Firm
- ☐ Q. Pharmacy
- ☐ R. Educational Institution
- ☐ S. Government Dept./Agency
- ☐ T. Policy or Resource Org.
- ☐ U. Policymaker
- ☐ V. Insurance Company
- ☐ W. Allied Health Professional
- ☐ X. Journalist
- ☐ Y. Drug Manufacturer
- ☐ Z. Library
- ☐ AA. Vendor/Supplier
- ☐ BB. Concerned Citizen
- ☐ CC. Other: (specify)

____

____

Place
First Class
Postage
Here

BOOK ORDER

HCS Publications
P.O. Box 781982
Dallas, TX 75378-1982